MW01196661

MAKING SPACE FOR THE DEAD

MAKING SPACE FOR THE DEAD

Catacombs, Cemeteries, and the Reimagining of Paris, 1780–1830

ERIN-MARIE LEGACEY

CORNELL UNIVERSITY PRESS
ITHACA AND LONDON

First published 2019 by Cornell University Press

Library of Congress Cataloging-in-Publication Data

Names: Legacey, Erin-Marie, 1979– author.
Title: Making space for the dead : catacombs, cemeteries, and the
   reimagining of Paris, 1780–1830 / Erin-Marie Legacey.
Description: Ithaca : Cornell University Press, 2019. | Includes
   bibliographical references and index.
Identifi ers: LCCN 2018042962 (print) | LCCN 2018046294 (ebook) |
   ISBN 9781501715617 (pdf) | ISBN 9781501715600 (epub/mobi) |
   ISBN 9781501715594 | ISBN 9781501715594 (cloth)
Subjects: LCSH: Burial—Social aspects—France—Paris—History—
   18th century. | Burial—Social aspects—France—Paris—History—
   19th century. | Pere-Lachaise (Cemetery : Paris, France)—History. |
   Catacombs—France—Paris—History. | Paris (France)—Social life and
   customs—18th century. | Paris (France)—Social life and customs—
   19th century. | France—History—Revolution, 1789–1799—Influence.
Classification: LCC GT3249.P37 (ebook) | LCC GT3249.P37 L44
   2019 (print) | DDC 393/.10944361—dc23
LC record available at https://lccn.loc.gov/2018042962

For my dad

CONTENTS

Illustrations

Acknowledgments

I visited Paris for the first time in the summer of 2006 to conduct preliminary research for what would eventually become this book. I am writing these acknowledgments twelve summers later. In the intervening years I have had the great privilege to spend countless hours in beautiful libraries and archives poring over historic texts; I have grown as a result of relationships with mentors and colleagues; and I have appreciated the unwavering support of friends and family. If it takes a village to raise a child, it takes at least two universities, three research libraries, dozens of workshops, seminars, and conference panels, and countless conversations to bring a book into the world. I am eternally grateful to everyone who helped me along the way.

My research and writing all reflect the influence of an exemplary group of mentors and advisors. I owe my first thanks to Bill Cormack, whose infectious enthusiasm inspired my love of the French Revolution when I was in my first year of university. His candid advice and encouragement also led me to graduate school, where I encountered so many brilliant scholars.

Harold Mah humored and honed my fascination with Jules Michelet—a strange nineteenth-century figure, whom I was delighted to resurrect for this book's conclusion. I cannot overstate how grateful I am to Sarah Maza for her elegant mentorship, consistent encouragement, and shining example. I hope Sarah sees her smart and stylish influence reflected in these pages. I am also very thankful to Suzanne Desan for teaching me how to write with conviction and confidence about the French Revolution. Tessie Liu offered invaluable advice and insight on earlier versions of this project. I am beyond lucky to have had such an accomplished group of women in my corner.

Many colleagues have kindly shared their time, their ideas, and their example with me as I worked on this book. Abby Swingen, Aliza Wong, and Kelly Wisecup all offered valuable advice and suggestions for my initial proposal, which no doubt helped this book find a great home. My fellow Texas Tech historians in our Junior Faculty Writing Group helped me sharpen the introduction and chapter 1, and I am grateful for their help: Emily Skidmore, Sarah Keyes, Angela Diaz, Catherine Franklin, Katie Moore, Ben Poole, Jake Baum, Matt Johnson, Rick Lutjens, Patrick Scharfe, and Dale Kretz. Lubbock has been a surprisingly easy place to live and work, and I feel very lucky to be a part of such a collegial and supportive history department. I finished up this book in the twelve months after my second daughter was born, often with a baby in my arms or by my side. I am fortunate to have had the support and encouragement of my colleagues during this time. I am particularly thankful for Sean Cunningham, a department chair who understands and appreciates the importance of work-life balance. I am also grateful to Elizabeth Sharpe and the Gender Equity Council at Texas Tech for working to build a more supportive and inclusive university. In particular, I appreciate the Women Faculty Writing Program: I crafted this book's introduction in the supportive silence of our weekly meetings.

I wrote the bulk of this book while in residence at the Newberry Library where I had the incredible good fortune of being the 2015–16 Andrew W. Mellon Foundation Fellow. While there, I was surrounded by a wonderfully interdisciplinary community of scholars. Our monthly fellows' seminars were a source of pleasure as well as edification, and I know my work benefited immeasurably as a result of my participation in them. I would especially like to thank the other long-term fellows for creating such a supportive and stimulating intellectual environment: Susan Gaylard, Kelly Wisecup, Miriam Thaggert, Kara Johnson, Christen Mucher, Chelsea Blackmore, Suparna Roychoudhury, Cynthia Wall, Kat Lecky, and Bill Brooks. Brad Hunt was a dedicated and energetic vice president for research and academic programs, and I appreciated his leadership and guidance. I also extend special thanks to one of the Newberry's scholars-in-residence, Christopher McKee, for his enthusiasm for my project and for generously offering to read drafts of chapters 3 and 4. It is perhaps a cliché, but my time at the Newberry was a genuinely transformative experience. Truly, there isn't a week that passes where I don't think fondly of my carrel on West Walton Street.

Friendships with smart and accomplished women have sustained me as I completed this book. In addition to those already mentioned, I want to thank Andreana Prichard, who has been by my side—in spirit, if not always in person—since the first day of graduate school. Julie Laut is a pillar of strength and wisdom who has taught me so much about balancing scholarship and motherhood. Emily Skidmore has been beyond generous with her advice since the day I met her and has set a sterling example that I strive to follow. I am also grateful for the online community of academic mothers (particularly those with babies born in 2017), whose advice, encouragement, good humor, strength, and honesty have been a daily source of inspiration and joy for me as this project neared completion.

Several organizations provided financial support for this book at various stages of its development. The Social Sciences and Humanities Council of Canada and the Graduate School at Northwestern University funded the initial research. As the project progressed and evolved, the History Department at Texas Tech University facilitated and supported additional research trips to Paris. Generous support from the Newberry Library and the Andrew W. Mellon Foundation provided me with the time, space, and resources to finally sit down and write. The office of the vice president for research at Texas Tech also provided much-appreciated financial support during my year in Chicago. The Humanities Center at Texas Tech generously helped with the acquisition of images and their copyrights.

When I began writing this book, I hoped that it would one day be published by Cornell University Press. At every stage of the publication process Cornell has exceeded my expectations. It has been a genuine pleasure to work with my editor, Mahinder Kingra. His patience, advice, and transparency turned a potentially daunting publication process into a truly enjoyable experience. I am grateful for the anonymous reviewers who read my manuscript and urged me to make my often-too-subtle arguments bolder and more pronounced. The final product is undoubtedly much sharper and more cohesive as a result of their thoughtful feedback. Thanks also to my production editor, Karen M. Laun, and my copyeditor, Jack Rummel, for helping push this book over the finish line.

Finally, but most elementally, I would like to thank my family, which has transformed in so many ways since this project began. After being my most ardent champion for over two decades, my father, Jamie, died several weeks before I began my Ph.D. program. In retrospect, however, it seems clear that he continued to exert great influence over my life and scholarship. I was not equipped to mourn his loss, so I bought a copy of Philippe Ariès's *The Hour of Our Death*, hoping to gain some historical perspective. Little did I know, it would launch me into more than a decade of my own research and writing. I hope that this book can serve in some small way as a memorial to his influence and example. My mother, Valerie, is one of the strongest women I have ever known: she and my brother, Brandon, have formed a solid bedrock of love and encouragement for my whole life. Thanks also to Joanie and Bob Poole for their unhesitating generosity and kindness.

My deepest gratitude is for Ben Poole, who supports and challenges me in the best of ways. His influence and ideas are laced throughout this book, because he has been with me on every step of this journey, from Evanston, to Paris, to Lubbock. I am truly fortunate to have such an informed and careful thinker by my side. Our two intrepid daughters, Maggie and Jane, inspire me every day with their bravery, love, and wild imaginations.

ABBREVIATIONS

AIF   Archives de l'Institut de France
AN   Archives Nationales de France
AP   Archives de Paris
BHVP   Bibliothèque Historique de la Ville de Paris
BNF   Bibliothèque Nationale de France
MMF   Annual Catalog of the Museum of French Monuments
        (1800–1821)

MAKING SPACE FOR THE DEAD

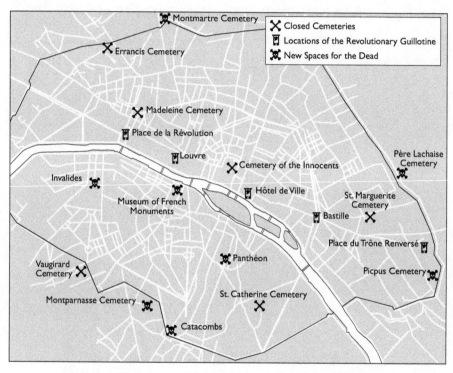

Spaces for the dead in Revolutionary Paris. Map prepared by Bill Nelson.

Introduction

The Revolution of the Dead

In December 1785, the dead moved from Paris's heart into what Victor Hugo would later call its intestines. Shadowy figures entered the city's oldest and largest cemetery, the Cemetery of the Holy Innocents, and began to dig. Inhabitants of neighboring buildings watched—some from their windows, and some from the street—as these men, working by torchlight, began the lugubrious and unprecedented process of emptying this historic burial space of its sacred contents. These city workers spent the next year digging human remains out of the cemetery's deep mass graves and collecting the millions of bones that had accumulated in charnel houses around its perimeter. They then systematically transported carts full of bones and human remains to an underground quarry on the city's southern periphery—a newly designated municipal ossuary that would soon be better known as the Paris Catacombs.[1]

This radical relocation was the culmination of a long campaign to end urban burial in the French capital. More specifically, it was the consequence of a 1780 royal ordinance that declared the Cemetery of the

Innocents to be an intolerable and illegal threat to the city, owing to the stinking vapors that constantly seeped from its muddy enclosure and endangered the health and well-being of anyone living in the neighborhood. The famous eighteenth-century chronicler of Parisian urban life, Louis-Sébastien Mercier, characterized the cemetery as an "immanent" danger, whose "cadaverous miasmas threatened to poison the atmosphere" of Paris. He further alleged that wine, milk, and bouillon served in the vicinity of the cemetery soured within hours and warned that the "cadaverous humidity" that clung to the nearby walls had lethal effects. "Yes," he explained, "to absentmindedly place one's hand against a wall impregnated with this moisture was to expose oneself to the effects of venom."[2] In this ancient space the dead were, quite literally, deadly.

Thirty years later C.-P. Arnaud, an architect and illustrator, walked through the gates of Paris's newest burial space, Père Lachaise Cemetery, and described it as unquestionably the most picturesque site in the capital. "This cemetery," he raved, "is nothing like the terrible and terrifying cemeteries that we used to see." Visitors to Père Lachaise had absolutely no need to fear exposure to any "putrid miasmas" or dangerous exhalations, he asserted. Instead, they could expect "a vast picturesque garden" filled with beautifully landscaped winding paths and alleyways. To further highlight the difference between Paris's old and new cemeteries, Arnaud noted that in the spring months, the air in Père Lachaise smelled of violets, lilacs, honeysuckle, and other flowering shrubs. He concluded his description of the new cemetery by promising that a visit to Père Lachaise would offer "the most interesting spectacle for the sensitive traveler," who would find, in the midst of tombs, "the most bucolic site" suitable for meditations on death, the beauty of nature, and other heady subjects.[3] In the span of a generation, Parisian spaces for the dead had completely transformed—both in reality and in the popular imagination—from deadly sources of contagion to delightful urban destinations.

This revolution in attitudes and design was not limited to Père Lachaise. Throughout the late eighteenth and early nineteenth centuries, Parisians could visit a succession of new urban spaces that contained, displayed, and commemorated the dead in new and exciting ways. These included well-known attractions, such as the Panthéon and the Catacombs, but also lesser-known sites such as a short-lived museum that brazenly displayed the tombs of all France's kings, from Dagobert to Louis XV. As the nineteenth-century historian Jules Michelet described this space, known as the Museum of French Monuments: "One could finally see France as she was, in her development, from century to century, and from man to man, from tomb to tomb."[4] Early nineteenth-century visitors to the Catacombs similarly treated the macabre subterranean space as a source of knowledge about themselves and their city. After touring the Catacombs in 1812, Thomas Détruisard encouraged others to similarly enter the so-called "Empire of Death" and bravely contemplate the "naked bones" on display. "They are of your brothers," he explained, "who yesterday knew life just as tomorrow, you will know death."[5] As comments like these demonstrate, Parisian spaces for the dead had undergone more than an aesthetic transformation since 1780. By the early nineteenth century, a new culture of the dead had developed in the city; one that reconciled Parisians to their burial sites as sources of collective identity rather than urban decay.

The backdrop of this transformation was, of course, the French Revolution. While revolutionaries inherited a burial crisis from the Old Regime—exemplified by the closing of the Cemetery of the Holy Innocents—they did significantly more than simply complete the work of their predecessors. Rather, revolutionary political culture irrevocably altered expectations about the role that the cemetery could (and should) play in the city of the future. This was the result of an unprecedentedly ambitious program to create a new France based on principles like justice, equality, liberty, and patriotic duty. In an about-face from earlier fears of contaminating urban cemeteries, revolutionary political culture elevated spaces and rituals associated with the dead. At its best, this manifested as Jacques-Louis David's spectacular public funerals for the assassinated "martyrs," Jean-Paul Marat and Louis-Michel le Peletier.[6] At its most notorious, the political power of the dead played out on the guillotine and in the infamous atheist cemeteries of 1793 that announced death to be "an eternal sleep." In each of these cases, radical revolutionary logic dictated that spaces for the dead were capable of doing considerably more than safely and securely containing human remains; they could also educate and improve the community of the living. As Jean-Baptiste Avril put it when pitching a proposal for comprehensive burial reform in 1794, a well-ordered cemetery culture would "sow the seeds of social and heroic virtues" among the population, ensure the happiness of future generations, and kindle the "sacred fire of patriotism" in all hearts.[7]

While many of the most controversial elements of revolutionary burial culture fell out of favor after the end of the Revolution's most radical phase (the Terror) in 1794, the state's underlying commitment persisted: to create new cemeteries that would safely contain the dead, while improving the social and moral character of the living. Indeed, this didacticism became even more pressing as the eighteenth century came to a close and legislators, moralists, and other interested individuals grew increasingly preoccupied with mitigating the social disorder that they considered inseparable from the cataclysm of revolution. In this anxious narrative, virtually everything that held Paris and Parisians together was in flux, including political tradition, a social hierarchy based on birth and privilege, and the authority and power of the Catholic Church. While constructing a new social and moral order seemed like an overwhelming task, establishing a coherent and well-ordered set of burial practices and spaces was comparatively straightforward. However, once they were actually built and open to the public in the first decade of the nineteenth century, Paris's new burial sites became remarkably complex social spaces that defied simple or consistent interpretations: one person's postmortem paradise could easily be another's shameless display of decadence. This book untangles the many overlapping—and sometimes conflicting—ways that Parisians used their new spaces for the dead to reimagine their collective identity in the wake of the Revolution. This vision for a new order was highly variable: depending on the venue and its audience, the France on display could be rigidly hierarchical, starkly egalitarian, or staunchly meritocratic. Similarly, it might recognize individual accomplishments, emphasize the communion of friendship, or celebrate a shared past. What these have in common, of course, is that they all represent attempts and opportunities to reorganize and restore a social order that seemed in pieces after the Revolution. This book argues that spaces for the dead—when they were first imagined, later built, and eventually used—provided a safe place to reassemble these pieces. The dead provided the glue.

Making Space for *the Dead*

The narrative that unfolds over the next five chapters is about the dead, but of course all stories about the dead are really about the living.

The interdisciplinary field of Death Studies has developed and expanded a great deal over the last few decades, but for the most part, scholars accept the basic tenet that a people's attitudes and practices related to the dead vividly illuminate their values, political structure, and social organization. An earlier generation of historians, such as Philippe Ariès and Michel Vovelle, demonstrated this phenomenon by focusing primarily on attitudes (*mentalités*) toward death. Despite drawing different conclusions (Vovelle was a Marxist and Ariès a self-proclaimed "anarchist of the right") both of these scholars agreed that a significant change in attitudes and behaviors toward the dead occurred in the eighteenth century.[8] They linked this transformation to bigger processes of modernization, including secularization, urbanization, and the rise of the middle-class family. Since the end of the twentieth century, however, historians such as Craig Koslofsky, Vanessa Harding, and most recently Thomas Laqueur have shifted the focus from attitudes to rituals, practices, and space.[9] Moreover, instead of interpreting death culture as something that reflects broader shifts, these scholars emphasize the power of the dead and their ability to help the living bring about (and process) radical change, particularly during times of flux. As Thomas Laqueur dramatically states in his 2015 book *The Work of the Dead*, "The work of the dead is to make culture and set the boundaries of our mortality."[10] This was especially the case during the era of the French Revolution with its underlying project of wholesale reinvention.

The experience of the French Revolution was instrumental in reshaping how Parisians considered the role of the dead in their city. Correspondingly, the dead offered revolutionaries opportunities to think through and experiment with the application of abstract values like equality, justice, and the radical presentism that accompanied the annihilation of the past. Many of the most iconic examples of revolutionary culture involve the display, discussion, or depiction of the dead. This is why Antoine de Baecque argued—somewhat provocatively—that by 1793 "the corpse" had become "the conceptual object that allow[ed] revolutionary politics to be thought out."[11] The dead became rallying points for a population in the midst of a revolution and looking to make sense of the changes taking place around them. An aristocrat was a frightening and nebulous bogeyman until he mounted the scaffold, when his destruction became a symbolic and purifying act, just as the blood of a "martyr" sanctified the revolutionary cause.[12] Similarly, as Joseph Clarke has demonstrated, the commemoration of the high-profile dead during the Revolution, whether through elaborate funeral processions or new civic spaces like the Panthéon, was a heavy handed (and ultimately unsuccessful) attempt to bind the population to the revolutionary state.[13] In short, the dead became powerful public figures and symbols during the Revolution—a significant departure from their Enlightenment-era role as a danger and a nuisance. At a moment when eighteenth-century Europeans were already in the process of reshaping their culture of the dead, as exemplified by the closing of the Cemetery of the Innocents in 1780, the startling events of the Revolution exploded and redirected that process.

This new role of the dead in the city was matched by an ambition to build worthy new cemeteries. As Richard Etlin has detailed, imaginatively conceived burial sites dated back to the end of the Old Regime, when Enlightenment architects drew up plans for elaborate city cemeteries that were never built.[14] The revolutionary spirit of reinvention breathed new life into this macabre civic project, which flourished again at the century's end. As this book articulates, the new spaces that appeared in Paris in the first decade of the nineteenth century gave shape to a new burial culture that was both a product of, and a reaction against, the experience of revolution. However, this book challenges some basic assumptions about the relationship between the Revolution and modern French burial culture. Most significantly, it complicates the notion that French cemeteries developed as highly polarized sites that reflected the tumultuous politics of the Revolution and its aftermath. Recent works have argued that in such a volatile context, cemeteries and death rituals became places for revolutionary reinvention, royalist expiation, and liberal resistance.[15] While a partisan tone certainly characterized the funerals and tombs of high-profile political and military figures, this divisiveness fades dramatically when we look beyond public spectacles of mourning and well-known gravesites. When early tourists to Père Lachaise Cemetery spied on their fellow Parisians sobbing at tombstones, they cried along with them. Underground in the Catacombs, visitors strongly identified with the "bona fide debris" of their predecessors on display. And in the ornate chambers of Paris's first history museum, disinterred tombs told the story of France's past, while poets buried in the backyard created a timeless community of sensitive souls. These stories all belie a reading in which nineteenth-century Parisian cemeteries were primarily ideologically charged sites that amplified the era's fractious political culture. In these new spaces where millions of Parisians lay buried, the pitched ideological battles of postrevolutionary France often gave way to a more benign spirit of concord.

These traces of communion rather than conflict all expand and challenge what we know about the aftermath of the Revolution. Historians often separate this era in two, with Napoleon Bonaparte serving as the barrier dividing the "post-Terror" period of 1795–1799 from the early nineteenth-century "postrevolutionary" era. Different narratives dominate each of these discrete phases. Since the publication of Bronislaw Baczko's *Comment sortir de la Terreur* in 1989, scholars of the Revolution have paid increased attention to the last five years of the eighteenth century as a time of great instability when French politics oscillated between left and right and the population sought to make sense of their recent violent past, whether through retributive violence, legal proceedings, or cathartic cultural practices.[16] By contrast, historians focusing primarily on the early nineteenth century emphasize the "search for stability" that characterized Bonaparte's project of domestic pacification and consolidation, which continued as the conciliatory *union et oubli* (unity and forgetting) of the Bourbon Restoration.[17] The story of Paris's new culture of the dead bridges these two periods and intertwines their dominant historical narratives. On one hand, it backdates the "search for stability" to 1795, when didactic proposals for burial reform really began to flourish, often as explicit solutions to the chaos and disorder that authors associated with the Revolution. On the other hand, it extends cathartic cultural practices well into the nineteenth century, when visitors to the Museum of French Monuments, the Catacombs, and Père Lachaise self-consciously reflected on the meaning and legacy of revolutionary violence.

In terms of its periodization, this book may feel elusive. It is at its core a book about reactions and responses to the French Revolution, but its chronology does not necessarily follow the "postrevolutionary" timeline. Moreover, although this book deals with three radically different political regimes, the rigid divisions between Revolution, Empire, and Restoration are much less significant than the common themes uniting this era, including social reorganization, cultural reinvention, and historical recalibration. This method of approaching the decades surrounding 1800 as a kind of continuum complements the work of other scholars who similarly interpret this era as a fruitful—if fraught—time that ultimately gave rise to many key features of modern French politics, society, and culture, from the bureaucratic and administrative state, to the bogeyman of the "bourgeoisie," to a distinctively nineteenth-century understanding of the self.[18] Like Paris's modern burial culture, the creation of all these institutions reveal a widespread desire for stable social spaces and categories in the wake of the Revolution.

But there were many paths to "stability" and many visions of what France could have been after the Revolution. The political side of this phenomenon is well known. In addition to the royalist, republican, and imperial programs, a diverse group of postrevolutionary intellectuals, administrators, and activists pitched myriad alternatives for France's political future, from Noel "Gracchus" Babeuf's communitarianism, to the liberalism associated with Germaine de Staël and Benjamin Constant, to the apocalyptic conservatism of Joseph de Maistre.[19] However, the aftermath of the Revolution was not limited to political theory. A parallel set of ideas about how to restructure the social world also circulated during this time. What kind of hierarchy (if any) would govern the nineteenth century? What kinds of shared values would form a solid foundation of *moeurs* to replace Catholic tradition? And what would provide the necessary social glue to bind individuals to each other, their nation, and their turbulent history?

Reformed burial spaces, both as proposed ideals and actually existing sites, quickly emerged as fecund environments where competing visions for social (re)organization circulated from the 1790s through the end of the Restoration. For example, throughout the 1790s intellectuals debated whether new cemeteries ought to be organized to reflect the "natural equality" of all citizens, or to showcase the reality of social hierarchies, whether based on wealth, birth, virtue, or merit. In practice, new spaces for the dead did all of the above: with its rows on rows of indistinguishable skulls, the Catacombs exemplified equality in death, while the short-lived Museum of French Monuments flipped Old Regime hierarchies by converting previously sacred royal tombs into artistic and historical curiosities. By contrast, Père Lachaise Cemetery quickly developed into a microcosm of the nineteenth-century Parisian economic pecking order, with its menu of options for burial and commemoration, ranging from

state-funded temporary burials for the indigent to permanent and lavishly adorned family mausoleums. However, within each of these new
sites, visitors found that they had ample space for reinterpretation. Not
everyone who toured the Catacombs "read" the bones in the same way,
and the opulence of Père Lachaise offended more than a few commentators who railed against the pretensions of Paris's middle-class upstarts.
While such variability frustrates any attempt at sweeping generalizations
about the meaning of these spaces, it may also be the key to understanding their power.

Making *Space* for the Dead

Theories of urban and social space underpin many of the claims in this
book, although they only make brief appearances in the text itself. Taking as my starting point Henri Lefebvre's famous assertion that "new social
relationships call for new spaces, and vice versa," I investigate the cemetery as a discrete "space" in the city.[20] In doing so, I follow the lead of other
scholars of this period who have demonstrated the different ways that Parisians understood and mapped their city after the Revolution. Throughout
the first third of the nineteenth century, Parisians, especially in the middle
class, displayed great interest in categorizing urban social space as a way
of making sense of the postrevolutionary world. In her analysis of Parisian
guidebooks before and after 1830, Victoria Thompson explained how early
nineteenth-century descriptions of the city overemphasized the differences
between (and homogeneity within) Parisian neighborhoods as a way of
imagining the postrevolutionary city as a "stable and harmonious whole"
in which clear social distinctions produced social stability.[21] Similarly,
Dominique Kalifa's work on the Parisian *bas-fonds* demonstrates how the
social imaginary of the dangerous criminal neighborhood, which relocated
repeatedly throughout the nineteenth century, often "turned out to be an
active force of cohesion and solidarity" in the modernizing city.[22] The desire
to create new city spaces specifically for foul smelling matter was an eigh-
teenth- and nineteenth-century project that went to the heart of these issues.
As Alain Corbin famously asserted, "It would be futile to analyze social ten-
sions and conflicts without accounting for the different kinds of sensibilities that decisively influence them."[23] Clearly, new ways of imagining and

describing their city helped Parisians articulate and address anxieties related to social reorganization after the Revolution.

However, cemeteries are qualitatively different from other kinds of urban space. They occupy a uniquely intermediary zone, which Michel Ragon has referred to as "a sort of antechamber, between this world and the next, a place of *passage.*"[24] As scholars like Victor Turner have long maintained, such liminality can be powerfully generative, particularly during times of radical transformation, when the possible outcome of that transformation is in flux.[25] The decades after 1789 were nothing if not radically transformative; this book investigates both the general liminality of this time period and the spaces it produced. For this I turn to Foucault, who also offered a theory—albeit less developed than Turner's—of liminality, specifically as it applies to space. His short essay, "Of Other Spaces," outlined the creative potential of alternative spaces that exist outside of (or in between) normative spaces. Indeed, the nineteenth-century cemetery was one of Foucault's most sustained examples of an "Other Space" (or heterotopia) that by the nineteenth century had become a kind of strange mirror of the regular city, where every living family had its dead analog.[26] Since Foucault, philosophers and geographers have debated the radical nature of heterotopias, particularly when discussing postindustrial Western cities. However, when thinking about France at the turn of the nineteenth century—a period that Foucault explicitly addressed in his original essay—many of his initial observations hold up. Particularly relevant is Foucault's assertion that heterotopias operate as "counter-sites capable of juxtaposing in a single real space, several sites that are in themselves incompatible."[27] This concept resonates particularly well with this book's overarching argument about the competing models of social organization that circulated in spaces for the dead. It was no accident that sites like Père Lachaise and the Paris Catacombs ended up being so intellectually productive: owing to their liminality (in both a geographic and conceptual sense) and their profound Otherness, they were almost predisposed to inspire multiple versions of the city they served.

But the usefulness of heterotopian theory does not end there. Foucault's claim that heterotopias "begin to function at full capacity when men arrive at a sort of absolute break with their traditional time" recalls another theme that runs throughout the book: that spaces for the dead repaired a crucial link to the past that was severed by the "absolute break" of 1789.[28] This book takes seriously the disorienting effect that the Revolution's proclaimed rupture in time had on the population. The dislocation caused by the Revolution was not just social, political, and cultural; it was also temporal. The (brief) adoption of a new calendar that restarted time on September 22, 1792, and the (even briefer) decimal clock were only the most idiosyncratic manifestations of a broader revolutionary repudiation of France's Catholic and royal past.[29] Accordingly, the "search for stability" that characterized France after the Revolution included a widespread desire to both reimagine and reconnect with the past that revolutionaries had so violently rejected. Scholars have long commented on the development of a modern historical sensibility around the turn of the nineteenth century; Stephen Bann even identified an "intense desire for history" as one of the defining features of the Romantic era.[30] The caesura of the French Revolution was central to this project, as Peter Fritzsche's work on the melancholy and nostalgia of the early nineteenth century has shown.[31] This book brings this widespread cultural phenomena into the graveyard by exploring the ways in which Parisians used spaces for the dead to make sense of an increasingly remote past.

Finally, it bears repeating that this is a story about Paris. Although many of the themes at work in this book characterize France as a whole during this time, it is explicitly a book about the capital. Between 1789 and 1795, Paris was the undisputed epicenter of the political and social Revolution, and after 1795 it was the site that administrators most ardently wanted to clean up and protect from further upheaval. Cemetery reform would eventually expand throughout the country (and far beyond), but it began in Paris and was influenced by Parisian events. Moreover, well before the eighteenth century, Paris had a special relationship with its burial spaces. As Vanessa Harding has noted in her comparative history of cemeteries in early modern Paris and London, the Cemetery of the Innocents had long been a symbol of civic identity, owing to the "sense of generations of Parisians buried there, [and] visibly present in the bones piled high in the attics of the surrounding *charniers*."[32] This was especially the case during times of strife, such as the wars of religion, when the cemetery (and who could be buried within its walls) became a powerful marker of Catholic identity. By the end of the eighteenth century, this identity no longer suited Paris, but the city's new spaces for the dead took up the mantle of representing the city and its new set of values, informed by the experience of revolution.

Making Space for the Dead

This book is organized into five roughly chronological chapters that tell the story of how and why Paris's new culture of the dead developed as it did between 1780 and 1830. It begins by demonstrating how the French Revolution dramatically altered the public's understanding and expectations of the dead. Although chapter 1 begins by reviewing the prerevolutionary reform movement, it ultimately argues that the Revolution dramatically intervened and influenced the course that these reforms took. While "Enlightened" reformers under the Old Regime expressed a pressing need for burial reform on the grounds of public health and hygiene, revolutionaries very quickly expanded the duties of France's future cemeteries. In the radical revolutionary imagination, cemeteries became much more than well-organized spaces to safely and securely contain the dead, they became veritable "schools of the living" to instruct and inspire future generations to virtuous behavior in both public and private. This didactic approach to death and commemoration mirrored the central role that the dead played in Revolutionary culture. Whether as guillotined enemies on the scaffold or revered martyrs paraded through the city, corpses were ubiquitous in republican political culture. However, the important role that the dead were supposed to play in the new republic was not matched by the reality of everyday life. Most Parisians who died during the revolutionary decade unceremoniously found their way into overflowing mass graves in ad hoc cemeteries. By the end of the Terror, individuals and communities rejected the dead in their city as more than a physical danger; they had also become disquieting reminders of the Revolution's failures.

Chapter 2 continues this discussion of cemeteries as spaces for moral and social reconstruction. It analyzes the range of ideas for burial reform that appeared between the end of the Terror and the beginning of the Napoleonic Empire (1794–1804). During this time the French state fell into a period of instability characterized by governmental corruption, oscillating politics, and economic collapse. In this climate of uncertainty, conversations about Paris's burial culture took on catastrophic tones. Critics observed widespread "indecency" and "indifference" toward the dead and interpreted it as a sign that the French moral and social character had been badly damaged by the experience of the Revolution. The solution, they all agreed, was a well-ordered set of burial practices. Relying primarily on a set of manuscript and printed proposals for burial reform, this chapter uncovers inventive designs that reconceptualized death and burial. With schemes that ranged from double cemeteries that divided the good from the wicked to mechanisms for turning human bones into inspiring glass sculptures, these reformers imagined a new burial culture for France that would be instrumental in constructing a postrevolutionary social and moral order that modeled good citizenship while unifying the fractured population around shared democratic values. However, this chapter also highlights the growing tension between the revolutionary legacies of liberty and equality. Cemetery reformers were split between those who believed burial sites should reflect and amplify "natural equality" and adherents to a more liberal view that emphasized each family's right to commemorate their dead as they wished. Although none of these proposed projects were implemented, they presaged the burial culture that would develop in the decade that followed.

When Napoleon Bonaparte took power, he was determined to reestablish order and stability in France. To accomplish this he embarked on a massive campaign of legal and civic reforms that included a complete overhaul of Parisian burial culture. Modern new sites to contain and commemorate the dead were essential to accomplishing this goal. Chapter 3 examines the most famous of these, Père Lachaise Cemetery, which opened to the public in 1804. It was the first modern cemetery in many ways: it was located outside of city walls; it featured ample greenery including flowering trees, bushes, and even a vegetable garden. Père Lachaise Cemetery also exemplified and resolved many of the contrasting visions of cemetery reform that had been circulating since the 1780s. Although the majority of Parisians were buried for free in the cemetery's semicommunal grave, they did have the option to purchase private burial plots. Approximately 18 percent of the cemetery's patrons paid for these private plots and embellished them according to their means. This hierarchy of burial resolved the decade-old question of how literally to interpret the "equality of death." However, it also quickly transformed the cemetery into a major tourist destination, which it remains to the present day. Early visitors to Père Lachaise described it as a unique liminal location that united the dead with the living and brought visitors together through affective acts of mourning. This cemetery sociability was evident on the many elaborately engraved tombstones on display, and in the pages of the guidebooks to Parisian cemeteries that began appearing shortly after Père Lachaise Cemetery opened its gates. These guidebooks are central to the narrative of this chapter, because they provide an emotional and physical map to the early history of Père Lachaise.

In chapter 4 the action moves underground to the Paris Catacombs. Although only accessible to the public beginning in 1809, the Catacombs originated in the last decade of the Old Regime, when the French state urgently needed a place to store millions of bones that were in the process of being exhumed from Paris's condemned urban cemeteries. The network of mining tunnels beneath the city offered an easy solution. City workers had been transferring bones into the ossuary for more than two decades when Napoleon Bonaparte ordered the department of mines to convert it into a public monument. The result was a unique underground space, lined from floor to ceiling with anonymous human bones. From 1809 until 1830, the Catacombs entertained almost-daily crowds of interested visitors, eager to descend the ninety steps into the "Empire of Death." Despite the popularity and cultural significance of the ossuary, historians of France have yet to engage in a sustained analysis of the Catacombs, likely owing to the lack of archival evidence. This chapter overcomes that problem by analyzing contemporary published descriptions in concert with the Catacombs' unpublished guest book, which from 1809 to 1813 collected signatures and comments from thousands of visitors. What emerges is an image of the Catacombs as a deeply conflicted, but unifying space that was capable of holding in balance many seemingly incompatible currents of French thought: religious and secular, conservative and liberal, superficial and profound. This chapter also introduces a new theme to the book—how spaces for the dead provided Parisians with a tangible link to a usable past. At a time when the relationship between the present and the past was continually being redefined, the dead provided an evocative physical remnant that eased this temporal crisis. In this vein, the Catacombs acted as a virtual portal into the city's past where visitors could surround themselves with ten generations of fellow Parisians.

The fifth and final chapter delves more deeply into the concept of the dead as history. It takes as its subject the long-extinct Museum of French Monuments, which stood on Paris's Left Bank as the nation's first history museum from 1793 to 1816. Alexandre Lenoir, an artist and revolutionary administrator, constructed the public museum out of thousands of sculpture fragments—most prominently, tombs—that had been confiscated from nationalized churches and the abandoned manor houses of émigré aristocrats. Lenoir also converted the museum's small courtyard into an "Elysian Garden" for the reburied remains of French cultural figures that he collected from throughout France, including Abélard and Héloïse, Molière, and Descartes. Although art historians have written extensively and thoughtfully about the Museum of French Monuments, they have generally overlooked the vital role of the dead in this space. Inside the museum, visitors could approach, observe, and touch a chronologically ordered procession of exhumed (and empty) royal tombs. By contrast, the Elysian Garden featured a syncretic display of newly constructed monuments for reburied intellectual figures. This chapter addresses the relationship between the interior and exterior of the museum and the very different narratives of French history that they conveyed to visitors. Through Lenoir's careful manipulation and placement of empty tombs, the history on display inside the museum's walls was complete and unchanging, whereas the Elysian Garden was a vibrant green space where the dead continued to inspire the living.

Several years after Louis-Sébastien Mercier made his vivid observations about the Old Regime's toxic cemeteries, he described the Museum of French Monuments in its earliest incarnation. "There, under my gaze, the accumulated centuries reached out their hand to me," he explained with excitement, immediately after noting how in the museum, "all ranks, all costumes, all crowns were beneath my feet."[33] Thus, although the museum differs significantly from the other spaces in this book in that it features the exceptional rather than the ordinary dead, it provides a useful capstone and overview of the broader phenomena under investigation in these pages. Paris's new spaces for the dead, whether beneath the city's streets, on its outer periphery, or at its very center, were all powerful spaces that transgressed seemingly impossible boundaries of time and mortality. They also confused conventional categories of social rank and political stripe and offered their visitors opportunities to try out new, alternative models for conceptualizing their city and nation. Between 1780 and 1830, spaces for the dead gave Parisians a chance to assert and assess their radical break with the past, to reconsider a new set of moeurs in the wake of that break, to reconnect with their fellow Parisians, both alive and dead, and to reimagine their past and its relationship to the present. Ultimately, restoring order to the dead in the city gave Parisians the opportunity to begin the difficult work of rebuilding their social world after the Revolution.

1

THE PROBLEM OF THE DEAD

In the spring of 1780 the scent of death crept into the basements of central Paris. More precisely, a row of buildings on rue de la Lingerie began to exude the distinctive and unwelcome smell of decomposing human remains. The street in question formed the western border of the city's oldest and largest burial space, the Cemetery of the Innocents, which had been in operation for more than five hundred years. On May 30 a resident of one of the afflicted houses, Monsieur Gravelot, lodged an official complaint with the state about the cadaverous odor, which he suspected to be the cause of his wife's recent illness. In response, the state dispatched Antoine-Alexis Cadet de Vaux, the city's recently appointed salubrity inspector, to investigate. In his report to the Royal Academy of Sciences later that year, Cadet de Vaux confirmed Gravelot's fears: poisonous gases had fully breached the barrier dividing Paris's living from its dead. In at least three houses along rue de la Lingerie, cemetery vapors had seeped into sub-basements and gradually made their way up to the ground floor. To underscore the urgency of the situation, Cadet de Vaux listed the various

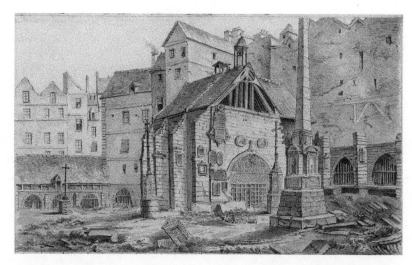

Figure 1.1. Claude-Louis Bernier, "The Cemetery of the Innocents along rue de la Lingerie in February 1786." Bibliothèque Nationale de France.

ailments that inhabitants of the quarter had been suffering as a consequence of their exposure, including respiratory ailments, delirium, "liver obstructions," and violent fits of vomiting. Although Cadet de Vaux embarked on a vigorous process to "demephitize" (*déméphitiser*) the basements, he remained convinced that the fix was temporary; the basements needed to be sealed off and the cemetery closed down.[1] The prerevolutionary state acted quickly and the centuries-old cemetery officially closed by the end of 1780, but Paris's burial problems were only just beginning.

When the Old Regime finally died after a long illness in the summer of 1789, it bequeathed a host of problems to its revolutionary successors. The most well known of these were the crippling fiscal and political crises that brought a centuries-old monarchy crashing down, but as the rue de la Lingerie incident illustrates French Revolutionaries also found themselves faced with a mounting burial crisis characterized by a shortage of spaces to safely and securely contain the dead. This problem afflicted the entire nation but it took on its most acute form in Paris, where a new Enlightenment attitude about the place of the dead in the city had the most influence.[2] For centuries Parisians had been burying their dead in graveyards located throughout the city, most of which were adjacent to parish churches. By the second half of the eighteenth century, the state, armed with scientific studies and expert testimony, like Cadet de Vaux's, decreed that this practice was dangerous to public health and contrary to reason. In practice, this meant that Paris's oldest and most problematic cemeteries were condemned, emptied out, and razed to the ground in the years before the Revolution. Although architects and urban planners proposed a range of new and improved urban burial spaces, reform had barely advanced out of the planning stage by the summer of 1789, when the Estates General met and irreversibly changed the course of history. Thus, in addition to higher-order projects, such as drafting a constitution and rethinking the tax system, early French Revolutionaries had to resolve the dirty business of where and how to bury their dead in the capital of their new nation.

Unsurprisingly, these revolutionaries were not content to simply continue the work of the Old Regime. As they sought to address their city's burial problem, Parisians during the Revolution began to rethink the relationship between the living and dead and explore the possibilities of a new burial culture that would be inseparable from the social and cultural reinvention of the era. In doing so, they dramatically changed the place of the dead in the capital. This process kept pace with the development of the Revolution: conversations about burial reform began in 1789 and accelerated at crucial moments when the dead caused problems and demanded attention, but it was not truly until the Revolution's most radical years, 1792–94, that a new approach to burial reform began to take shape, characterized by inventive new types of republican burial spaces. However, this revolutionary intervention also introduced a whole new set of problems that would spill over into the nineteenth century. In addition to the logistical issues inherited from the Old Regime, such as the location and layout of new cemeteries, revolutionaries added conceptual concerns, including the role of religion, the tension between equality and hierarchy, and the place of the past in Paris's new spaces for the dead.

Historians have generally glossed over the role that cemetery and burial reform played in the republican cultural project. This is probably because none of the planned or proposed revolutionary spaces for the dead were actually built, with the very notable exception of the Panthéon, which has certainly received its share of attention and analysis.[3] Scholars interested in the place of the dead during this time have tended to focus on elaborate funeral festivals for exceptional revolutionaries and the ongoing spectacle of public violence.[4] When addressing ordinary cemeteries during the

Revolution, their discussion is usually limited to passing comments about de-Christianization and notorious atheist cemetery signage announcing death to be "the eternal sleep." However, the debate about cemetery reform that began at the end of the Old Regime persisted throughout the Revolution, shifting and transforming with the radicalization of political culture. The Panthéon, republican funerals, and de-Christianization all contributed to this conversation, but they did not make up the whole story. Focusing only on accomplished projects elides other powerful ideas that were taking root during the Revolution about the role that the cemetery could play in the city, including a manifestation of social equality, a temporal link between the past and the present, and a site that powerfully bound citizens to each other and to their *patrie.*

Public Health and Cemeteries in the Old Regime

Prior to the 1780s, most Parisians buried their dead in the city, usually in a mass grave adjacent to their parish church. Although this kind of urban interment had been prohibited during the early Christian era for reasons of salubrity, by the ninth century the church began making exceptions for bishops, abbots, and priests who wished to be buried on church grounds. This paved the way for civilian church burial, which expanded during the medieval and early modern period, so that by the eighteenth century virtually all Parisians were buried in one of the city's thirty-two churchyard burial spaces.[5] However, the largest and oldest of the city's burial sites, the Cemetery of the Holy Innocents, followed a slightly different model. Although it was owned by a religious community, Innocents was less of a church graveyard than a public and civic cemetery, because so many of the capital's neighborhoods and institutions had the right to bury their dead in it, including eighteen parishes, two hospitals, and the city morgue. Innocents was also notable for its size and age: locals had been burying their dead in the area since antiquity, but during the reign of Philippe II (r. 1180–1223) the burial site was expanded to occupy a huge swath of walled-in urban space on the city's right bank, adjacent to the les Halles marketplace. By the middle of the eighteenth century, one-tenth of the city's dead (approximately eighteen hundred people) found their way into Innocents each year.[6] Perhaps owing to its size and age,

Innocents had long been associated with the city as a whole, as opposed to a particular neighborhood, parish, or population group, as smaller parish graveyards were. Indeed, throughout the early modern period, and especially during moments of strife, such as the wars of religion, city dwellers widely regarded Innocents as a powerful symbol of Parisian (Catholic) identity.[7]

Yet in the decades before the French Revolution, a new narrative began to supplant the earlier mythology of Innocents and urban burial in general. While burial on church property had long been standard, during the eighteenth century, a powerful scientific critique of this practice gained traction in educated circles. For centuries, physicians and natural philosophers had cautioned against the menace of bodily decay in the capital, citing miasmic theory. Eighteenth-century medical experts added legitimacy to this long-held concern with evidence culled from experimentation.[8] This began in 1737 when the Parlement of Paris sponsored a medical inquiry to explore the relationship between cemeteries and public health. Two doctors from the Hôtel-Dieu hospital and one local apothecary oversaw the study. The resulting report was neither published nor widely circulated, and it focused less on the need to eliminate urban burial, than on recommendations on how to improve the salubrity of the cemetery, including a soil transplant from a much newer nearby cemetery.[9] Three decades later, public complaints about Parisian cemeteries continued to accumulate, triggering a new report in 1763 about the sorry state of cemeteries in the capital. This detailed report on the status of each of the city's cemeteries described mass graves that stayed open for months at a time, graveyards that contained so many corpses that the level of the soil was above that of the surrounding houses, and bones stacked above the rafters in churches whose charnel houses were full. The report also vividly noted that "the burials that take place in Paris are thickening the air" and surmised that "the cadavers buried beneath our feet" were the source of "otherwise mysterious illnesses" affecting city dwellers.[10]

In response to these widespread fears, the Parlement of Paris issued an ordinance in 1765 that condemned church burial for almost everyone and strongly suggested that all burials after January first of the new year take place in large cemeteries that would eventually be built outside of the city walls.[11] This measure pleased educated reformers but met with hostility throughout the country, especially in ecclesiastical circles. The curates of

Paris, in particular, produced a long and detailed refutation of the decree, arguing that "the people" would suffer if traditional churchyard cemeteries were shut down, because "the very poorest do their best to have the bodies of their loved ones taken from [the hospital] Hôtel-Dieu to [the Cemetery of the] Innocents."[12] While the curates' objections may have been motivated by economic as much as altruistic concerns (since they would have been the ones to foot the bill for these new cemeteries), they did raise an important point when they invoked popular attachment to the city's ancient burial grounds.[13] While many Parisians, particularly among the educated elite, had come to interpret and condemn urban cemeteries as dangerous, the attitudes of the working poor toward their cemeteries were less clearly defined. As one Parisian journalist noted at the time, many Parisians had a natural and sentimental attachment to the place where their parents were buried.[14] The general outcry against the 1765 ordinance proved fatal, and none of the laws were enforced.

It took the calamity at the rue de la Lingerie in 1780 to finally bring about real and lasting change. In his report before the Royal Academy of Sciences, Antoine Alexandre Cadet de Vaux explained that the air in Innocents was as infected and insalubrious as in the city's most notorious hospitals. However, at the end of this otherwise scathing report, Cadet de Vaux imagined a better Paris, one in which everyone breathed cleaner air, where future generations would be spared the effects of "cadaverous exhalations," and where the dead would "finally stop troubling the living."[15] Louis XVI's government responded with a definitive decree that immediately ordered Innocents—and eventually all urban cemeteries— permanently closed. As a writer for the *Journal de Paris* noted later that year, only the ignorant or those acting in bad faith could possibly refute the danger that the dead posed to the living.[16]

For five years, Innocents sat quiet and unused until mass exhumations of the cemetery began in December 1785. It took six months of constant work to fully excavate the cemetery and remove more than twenty thousand cadavers. In Louis-Sébastien Mercier's opinion, the excavation process was ominous, fascinating, and long overdue.[17] He described a nocturnal scene in which city workers appeared as ghostly shadows, systematically dismantling funerary structures and pulling human remains out of mass graves and where the local residents of the area "woke up and rose from their beds, some came to their windows, half-dressed; others came down into the street." The whole neighborhood, he explained, rushed to witness the historic event, with youth and beauty standing in stark contrast with "this debris of the dead!"[18] Similarly, the report of the Royal Medical Society described the excavation as an "important and lugubrious" process.[19] Although authors of the report noted the historic and religious significance of the Cemetery of the Innocents, they spent most of the report detailing the various states of decomposition and mummification that they observed among the disinterred cadavers.[20] Both of these accounts demonstrate how significantly the imagined place of the cemetery had changed over the course of the eighteenth century. Far from being a powerful site of religious and urban identity, the historic burial ground was reduced to a morbid curiosity, albeit one rich with scientific knowledge.

Resolving the crisis at the Cemetery of the Innocents was not the end of Paris's cemetery problems. Although Innocents was certainly the most notorious of the city's "infected" cemeteries, it was not the only one, and increasingly throughout the 1780s residents of various neighborhoods in Paris petitioned the state to take similarly dramatic action toward their (much maligned) parish graveyards. For example, the inhabitants of St. Eustache parish in Montmartre lodged several detailed complaints in August and September 1786 to Guillaume-François-Louis Joly de Fleury, the Procurator General of Paris in which they vividly described their parish cemetery "vomiting forth an unbearable stench" that caused great suffering throughout the neighborhood.[21] Adding insult to injury, the petitioners noted that when the Cemetery of the Innocents was emptied out in January 1786, the convoys of human remains traipsed directly through their neighborhood for two nights in a row, trailing "infected air" and leaving bits and pieces of human remains in their wake. By the summer, entire families were forced to relocate to avoid the quarter's dangerous air, no one wanted to visit the area, and cadaverous exhalations regularly drove workers to abandon their projects midstream. The danger of a medical epidemic, they explained, was imminent. More than thirty inhabitants signed the longest and most detailed petition against the Saint-Eustache Cemetery.[22] These particular complaints were initially dismissed by the state as the self-interested machinations of a neighborhood rabble-rouser, but in 1787 Saint-Eustache became the second Parisian cemetery, after Innocents, to be closed down and emptied out.

By the summer of 1789, when the Estates General met and unexpectedly transformed Paris into a revolutionary city, only a third additional parish cemetery had been condemned and emptied of its contents (Saint-Étienne-des-Grès). Yet reform was certainly underway and inventive proposals for burial began appearing in state offices. These ranged from vague assertions about the need to construct four large suburban cemeteries, to a detailed and specific design for a single colossal "catacomb" that would serve the entire city.[23] Although it took a few years to gain momentum, Revolutionaries eagerly took up the mantle of cemetery reform, which they quickly tailored to meet the specific needs and interests of the new state.

The Cemetery and the Early Revolution

Although a new understanding of the cemetery's place in the city would eventually develop, the discourse of salubrity continued to dominate conversations about burial reform during the early months of the French Revolution. Individuals concerned with urban burial generally tended to pitch their arguments in the language of public health and hygiene, drawing on generations of scientific research and advice. For example, as early as November 1789 a curate from Saint-André-des-Arts in Paris, M. Desbois de Rochefort, reminded the newly created National Assembly to continue and expand the prior regime's work of burial reform. His statement leaned heavily on a public health argument, demanding an end to burials inside of the city.[24] However, several months later in a letter to the national daily newspaper, the *Moniteur universel*, Desbois abandoned these familiar arguments and turned instead to the moral and social aspects of cemetery reform. This shift is not entirely surprising if one accepts Thomas Laqueur's argument that the public health argument for burial reform was an Enlightenment-era disguise for anticlericals looking to wrest control of the dead from the Catholic Church.[25] By the time that Desbois made his second appeal for burial reform, that task was well underway.

The first year of Revolution brought unprecedented change to the city, which Desbois's second appeal directly addressed. As a member of the former first estate (the Catholic Church), he was particularly interested in the implications of the revolutionary state assuming control over many of the church's prior functions. Specifically, Desbois was worried about how the administrative reorganization of the city—from twenty-one quarters to sixty political sections—would affect burial. If each new section did not contain a cemetery of its own, he cautioned, Paris's already precarious burial culture might tip into chaos, with too much of the population vying for the same burial space. However, Desbois was also interested in how the Revolution's recent acquisition of church property might afford new possibilities for burial reform. After nationalizing all church property in November 1789, the revolutionaries found themselves in possession of unprecedented territorial and material wealth, including a vast number of mausolea and funerary sculptures. Desbois reasoned that rural property in particular provided the perfect opportunity for cemetery construction. He further proposed that all of the state's newly acquired pieces of funerary art would be an excellent (and appropriate) way to outfit these new sites.[26] Desbois's shift in tone reveals both his anxiety over the urgency of burial reform and his excitement about the potential for real and productive change after 1789.

Despite these early rumblings, a national conversation about burial reform did not truly begin to take shape until the spring of 1791. A flurry of newspaper letters, pamphlets, and proposals began to appear in April and May, as a direct consequence of the death of one of the Revolution's early heroes, Honoré Gabriel Riqueti, comte de Mirabeau. Scholars have emphasized the political significance and many unique aspects of Mirabeau's death and commemoration, such as his very public autopsy and his elaborate state funeral.[27] However, this somber event and the publicity surrounding it also provide an excellent opportunity to gauge attitudes and ideas about the place of the dead in the revolutionary city at a crucial moment. By the spring of 1791, the first era of the Revolution seemed to be coming to a close: the new constitution was almost complete and most of the major domestic and international crises that would soon plague France were months away, including the Champ de Mars Massacre, the royal family's attempt to flee the country, and the beginning of the war with other European powers. This was still a time of relative optimism about the Revolution's success and potential. In this climate of hope, discussions about what to do with the dead body of one of the nation's most cherished legislators quickly gave rise to broader and more comprehensive conversations about what a revolutionary burial culture might to look like.

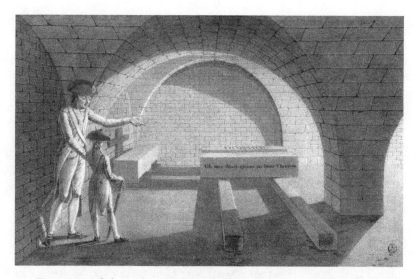

Figure 1.2. A father and son at the tomb of Mirabeau in the Panthéon, 1791.
Bibliothèque Nationale de France.

Before his death Mirabeau had specifically requested for his corpse to be transported to the nearby suburban community of Argenteuil where it could be buried with the rest of his ancestors. Despite his wishes, there was an immediate and widespread demand to keep Mirabeau's corpse in the capital permanently. As the renowned architect Antoine-Laurent-Thomas Vaudoyer argued less than a week after Mirabeau's death, Mirabeau's love of family was admirable, but when it came down to it, he was a man of the patrie and as such, he belonged to the nation. The state thus owed Mirabeau special honors after death, but more to the point, it had an opportunity, perhaps even an obligation, to commemorate and display Mirabeau's remains in the most useful way possible. Two days after his death, Mirabeau was celebrated with an elaborate revolutionary state funeral and his body was laid to rest in the former church of Sainte Geneviève, remodeled and renamed as the French "Panthéon." His was the inaugural corpse in this new institution dedicated to preserving the bodies and memories of the nation's great men—a rather heavy-handed attempt to craft a stable moral and intellectual heritage for the fledgling state.[28]

Despite Mirabeau's almost instantaneous "pantheonization," politicians, artists, architects, and other interested citizens continued to debate the issue throughout April. Vaudoyer was particularly vehement in his opposition to the Panthéon in general. Enclosing the illustrious dead in a dark underground temple was an unfortunate waste of their social potential, he explained. To support this claim, he noted that very few Parisians had ever visited dead military heroes entombed in Les Invalides or seen Cardinal Richelieu's tomb, which had laid in the Sorbonne since his death in 1642.[29] As an alternative to such stodgy commemorative practices, Vaudoyer recommended that the state convert one of Paris's well-traveled streets, such as the Champs-Elysées, into an open-air cemetery for its dead heroes, similar to Rome's Appian Way. He argued that the already-illustrious boulevard would become even more impressive if it were lined on both sides by simple allegorical monuments and the buried remains of France's greatest and most virtuous citizens, including Mirabeau, Voltaire, and Rousseau.[30] Vaudoyer dismissed competing ideas, which included burying Mirabeau beneath the altar to the fatherland on the symbolic Champ de Mars (where the Eiffel tower now stands). Burying the dead on a well-traveled street guaranteed that France's great men would be visited daily by "a thousand Frenchmen and just as many foreigners" who would spill their tears and return home committed to imitating the virtues and good behavior of the dead. He further imagined fathers with their sons and tutors with their students, all sharing valuable lessons as they strolled along Paris's new "Honor Way."[31]

Antoine Quatremère de Quincy, the architect who actually oversaw the conversion of the church of Sainte Geneviève into the Panthéon, opposed Vaudoyer's open-air scheme, but he agreed with his colleague's assessment that new spaces for the dead needed to be beautiful, inspiring, and welcoming to visitors.[32] He argued that the overwhelming tone of a burial space—whether for the illustrious or ordinary citizens of France—needed to be peaceful and soothing instead of frightening and macabre. Gothic images of skulls, skeletons, or "other infantile ridiculousness" had no place in a modern cemetery where the objective was not to frighten through memento mori but to educate and regenerate through example. This was an explicit and deliberate rejection of the type of memento mori that had famously characterized medieval and early modern spaces like the Cemetery of the Innocents (see figure 1.3). Whatever form they were destined to take, France's new cemeteries needed to welcome and invite citizens, rather than "repulsing" them. Cemeteries that avoided the

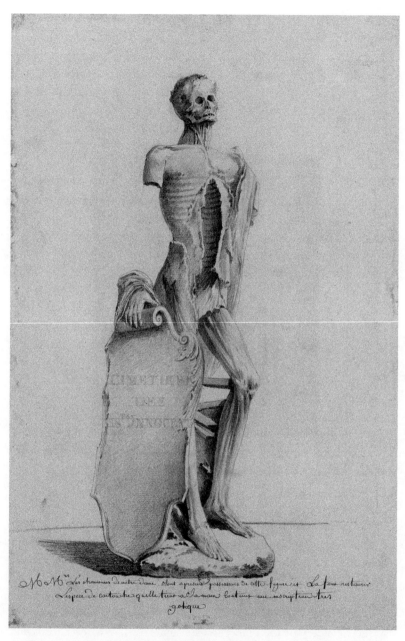

Figure 1.3. Claude-Louis Bernier, "The Statue of Death in the Cemetery of the Innocents," 1786. Bibliothèque Nationale de France.

"repugnant" images of Old Regime graveyards opened up new possibilities for public instruction and the cultivation of a sensitive, civic-minded population. Of course, this hostility toward the conventional aesthetic of the graveyard signaled more than an optimistic shift in tone; it was also at the heart of the increasingly tense relationship between the revolutionary state and the Catholic Church.

Secularization was one of the most significant—and contentious—ways in which revolutionaries transformed Parisian burial culture. In May 1791, M. Treilhard presented a petition before the National Assembly on behalf of Parisians requesting a law that would bring burial, along with marriage and baptism, under civil rather than ecclesiastical administration. His motion led to "long and tumultuous debates" in the assembly, which reflected the increasingly tense relationship between the revolutionary state and the Catholic Church.[33] This type of project was perfectly in line with the Revolution's broader program to curb the political influence of the church and to bring its administration under the umbrella of the state. For some, the conversation about cemetery reform was at the very heart of these negotiations. In 1792 Charles-Alexandre de Moy, an ardent revolutionary and priest outlined his vision for ideal church-state cohabitation. He dedicated eleven out of twenty-four chapters to the management of the dead in his pamphlet about the role of religion in a free nation, *Accord de la religion et des cultes chez une nation libre.* His theories about cemetery and burial management reflect his overarching position that while "perfect equilibrium" between religion and politics ought to be the end goal, the needs and responsibilities of individuals as members of a society must ultimately take precedence over their faith as individuals. To this end, he explained that priests had dominion over the souls of the dead, but not their bodies, and as such they had no right to care for, transport, or bury the dead. Religious ceremonies and rituals wrenched the dead from their friends and family, he explained, and severed a vital link that connected all members of society to one another. In this undesirable scenario, he imagined society shamefully turning its back on the dead and neglecting their duties. Instead, he emphasized that after a lifetime of service and participation, citizens deserved to be valued, honored, and commemorated by their peers.[34]

To Moy, establishing unique and relatively isolated burial spaces was a crucial task for society to fulfill its obligation to the dead. Such designated sites would naturally prevent pestilential vapors from infecting the living, but they would also ward against abuses of the dead. Expanding on this idea, he noted how the convention of burying the dead in highly accessible spaces in the middle of cities inevitably devalued burial grounds because it converted them into public passageways, where countless city dwellers trampled over the dead each day without giving them a second thought. Moreover, he despaired that legions of children used urban cemeteries as arenas for their turbulent games and feuds.[35] Although Christine Métayer has shown that the Parisian community that developed around a space like the Cemetery of the Innocents was a vibrant neighborhood in its own right, for Moy, multiuse cemeteries were as indecent as putrid miasmas.[36] Unsurprisingly, Moy also opposed macabre signs of death designed to frighten the living, including somber music and the iconography of bones. He was particularly opposed to the image of a scythe-wielding skeleton, which he found ridiculous and anatomically impossible, since skeletons without any muscle on them would not be able to stand upright, let alone lift a heavy farming implement.[37] Instead, Moy recommended planting cemeteries with evergreens, flowers, and other pleasant fixtures that would draw people to the cemetery where they could maintain relationships with their dead friends and family. Of course, this connection was more than personal. In new, secular cemeteries, he explained "the memory of those who have left us will stay with us, and their precious memory will always unite us to the motherland [*mère-patrie*]."[38] Well-planted cemeteries would cultivate a vital link between the grave and society.

During this first moderate phase of the Revolution engaged citizens increasingly invested the dead and their spaces with great social and political power. Even before the violent spectacle of the Terror, Parisian architects, writers, and politicians began thinking seriously about the dead as a powerful but untapped fount for public instruction and social cohesion: the dead could provide models of civic virtue and act as a bridge uniting past and present. This historical work was particularly valuable given the revolutionaries' enthusiasm for instituting a "radical break" with the past. However, investing so much power in cemeteries did not always work to the advantage of the dead, as the events of 1792 and 1793 would soon show. Just as the new state needed new civic heroes, so too did it need villains.

Digging Up the Dead during the Terror

As domestic and international politics radicalized during the late summer of 1792, conversations and concerns about the place of the dead in Paris grew accordingly extreme. In Paris, a successful insurrection on August 10 overthrew the elected government and nullified the new constitution. Louis XVI was arrested for treason and France made the abrupt and historic transition from constitutional monarchy to republic. Moreover, the nation had been officially at war with Austria and Prussia since April and by the early days of September it had yet to win any major battles. When the Prussian Army began to advance into France, rumors circulated that if the enemy invaded the capital, the thousands of prisoners in Paris would rise up against their revolutionary jailers. Fearful of this impending prison plot, crowds of armed civilians and national guardsmen rushed to the city's prisons, established ad hoc tribunals, and summarily executed roughly half of the city's prisoners—upwards of twelve hundred individuals. These bloody events soon became known as the "September Massacres," and for generations historians have used these notorious days as a signifier of the Revolution's slide toward Terror. This moment of heightened tension in the capital also led to a shift in behaviors and ideas about the place of the dead in the revolutionary city.

On a practical level, the September Massacres created the temporary problem of how and where to dispose of so many dead bodies. An eighteen-year-old visitor to the city from Bordeaux, Edmond Géraud, later described how "at every step you can see the hideous and bloody remains of mutilated bodies in open graves. I saw for my part, seven of these graves, filled with more corpses than they could hold; the horrifying carts left trails of blood in their wake; the image of death and of the massacre was present everywhere and in the most terrifying ways."[39] The accepted narrative seems to be that by the second week of September, the piles of corpses that had been rotting in prison courtyards were gradually transported to "pits" on the outskirts of Paris and covered with quicklime to hasten decomposition.[40] This makes it seem as though the September corpses simply vanished on the edges of the city, leaving no permanent physical trace behind. In fact, the problematic corpses found their way to five separate burial spaces in the city, including four already-full public cemeteries and the subterranean ossuary that locals had taken to calling the "Paris Catacombs," where they would enjoy a long afterlife as objects of fascination for tourists and Parisians alike. However, just as the massacred dead were being hurried out of view, the city's long dead also came under attack.

On the last day of the September Massacres, angry crowds turned their sights from the city's prisons to its churchyards. As citizen Bazire, speaking on behalf of a neighborhood surveillance committee, described it, on the night of September 7 "a number of citizens driven by foolhardy zeal" had taken it on themselves to invade several of the city's churches to exhume the dead clergymen and Aristocrats who were buried there. The alleged goal of these disinterments was to contribute to the nation, by securing precious metals and jewels or materials that could benefit the war effort, such as lead, which could melted down and repurposed as bullets.[41] It is difficult to ignore the resonance of this act: ardent revolutionaries digging up the elite of the Old Regime and scavenging anything of value from their bones for the benefit of the Revolution and its war against the monarchies of Europe. This opportunity for symbolic acts of destruction was certainly not lost on contemporaries. Indeed, when Ponce Denis Échouard Lebrun wrote a "patriotic ode" about the radical events of the fall of 1792, he described a desire to tear Charles IX from his two hundred-year-old tomb. He also passionately called for patriots to "reject the bones of the despots," smash their coffins, and purge their cadavers from the patrie.[42] The ode was so well received that it appeared in the national newspaper in early February 1793.

Lebrun was not the only advocate for the destruction of royal tombs. In early January 1793 Louis Prudhomme made a similar statement in his weekly newspaper *Les Révolutions de Paris*, when he explicitly called for the disinterment and destruction of France's dead kings:

> While we are in the process of erasing all vestiges of royalty, how is it that the impure remains of our kings continue to lay intact in the caves beneath the former Saint-Denis abbey? We have helped ourselves to the effigy of all of our despots; not a single one was pardoned. Stone, marble, bronze, nothing was saved. Equestrian or pedestrian statues, busts, bas-reliefs, paintings, drawings, engravings, every image of the kings was removed from our view, and yet we put up with their relics, preciously conserved in lead tombs, and insulting to the memory of so many good citizens who died for the patrie and for liberty without ever receiving the honor of a burial![43]

Several months later, on July 31, 1793, the radical journalist and elected member of national government, Bertrand Barère, made an identical appeal for the destruction of France's royal tombs, which all lay in Saint-Denis Abbey, several kilometers north of Paris. For centuries, Saint-Denis had sheltered the entombed remains of French royalty, from Dagobert (d. 638) to Louis XV (d. 1774). Barère explained that in the summer of 1793, when France was at war with multiple hereditary monarchies, including Austria, Prussia, and England, it was vital for France to reiterate its wholesale rejection of the Old Regime. He announced that "the powerful hand of the Republic" had a duty to "mercilessly erase" royal epitaphs and "demolish" the mausoleums of the past. To amplify its significance, Barère suggested that this mass exhumation take place on August 10, 1793, which was the one-year anniversary of the insurrection that overthrew the monarchy and led to the founding of the republic. What better way to commemorate the dethronement and arrest of France's last king, Louis XVI, than by desecrating the remains of his predecessors and melting down the fragments of their broken tombs to make cannon balls and bullets for the republic?[44]

The National Convention immediately approved Barère's recommendation and ordered the destruction of the royal tombs in honor of August 10. They named a former Benedictine monk, Dom Germain Poirier, to observe and report on the destruction process.[45] From August 6 to 8, Poirier watched as zealous republicans disinterred fifty-one tombs, dating from the seventh through fifteenth centuries. As revolutionaries extracted the tombs from the ground, they took care to set aside anything of value, including jewels or precious metals. Lead coffins and adornments were dispatched to the national foundry. As for the human remains: they were hastily buried in an unmarked mass grave behind the church. The local inhabitants of Saint-Denis—or Françiade as the commune was briefly known during the Revolution—continued the symbolic work of this recycling project. They collected pieces of the broken tombs and piled them up to construct a kind of secular and patriotic grotto that prominently featured large busts of the Revolution's two most famous martyrs, Jean-Paul Marat and Louis-Michel le Peletier. An eyewitness later described how decorative marble was repurposed into ceiling vaults while bits of royal sculpture were repurposed as pediments in "this bizarre monument to Liberty."[46] Weeks earlier, this material had protected the bodies of France's oldest kings, now it propped up the secular gods of the new republic.

This powerful act of desacralization and reinscription continued several months later in October when the state dispatched a new delegation to continue the work that had begun in August. From October 12 until October 25, the remaining members of the entombed monarchy, from Henri IV to Louis XV were systematically exhumed, examined, and discarded. However, these monarchs suffered further indignities than their predecessors had in August. For example, Henri IV clothed in his funeral shroud, was removed from his coffin and publicly displayed in the lower chapel of the cathedral for two days until he was thrown into a large mass grave (see figure 1.4). Eyewitness testimony from the exhumation described Henri IV's corpse as a perfectly preserved mummy, whose skull was filled with seventeenth-century aromatics that continued to exude an almost intolerably strong scent almost two hundred years after his death. By the same account, an unnamed revolutionary soldier who was present

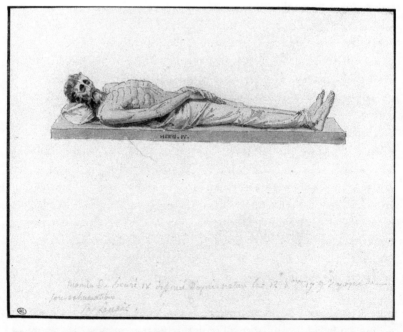

Figure 1.4. Alexandre Lenoir, "The Remains of Henri IV, Exhumed from His Tomb in 1793." Musée du Louvre, RMN-Grand Palais/Art Resource NY.

during the exhumation was so excited to be in Henri IV's presence that he used his saber to cut a lock of his red beard, which he then placed under his nose, announcing, "Now I am sure to vanquish France's enemies, onwards to victory!" Louis XIV's body was allegedly similarly well preserved, but ironically, the sun king had turned an inky shade of black since his death.[47]

Such vivid descriptions of the exhumation accentuated the important historical work that revolutionaries accomplished at Saint-Denis. The destruction of the royal tombs was only one component of a broader campaign to "destroy all signs of feudalism" in France, in an attempt to create a visible and lasting break with the Old Regime. The somatic cataloging and description of the royal corpses—of their appearance, texture, and smell—was every bit as revolutionary as their destruction.[48] When Louis XV's coffin was opened on October 16, 1793, an eyewitness described how his skin was white, his nose violet, and his buttocks as pink as a newborn baby's. The body was quickly thrown in the communal grave and covered with quicklime. This corporeal destruction— in both text and reality—had obvious ties to the execution of the royal couple in 1793. Artists produced countless replications of the image of Louis XVI, headless and on the scaffold.[49] The revolutionaries were well aware of this rapport, indeed they had arranged this second round of royal exhumations to coincide with Marie Antoinette's execution on October 16. To this end, Louis XV's body was disinterred on the same day, and possibly even at the same hour that his granddaughter-in-law lost her head in Paris.[50]

Throughout 1793, revolutionaries continued to exhume and destroy historic tombs and corpses in the capital. In November a group of representatives from the Paris Commune extracted several tombs from the fifteenth-century church, Saint-Étienne-du-Mont. When they opened the tombs they were excited to find pearls, diamonds, and other precious goods worth almost twenty-four thousand livres. After delivering a very detailed report about this event, and removing anything of material value, the general council of the Paris Commune made the bold (but not surprising) decision to publicly burn all of the bones and clothing that remained from the historic tombs. This bonfire, they explained, would serve a valuable expiatory service for the republic by consuming the remains of the aristocracy along with the symbols of their luxury and idleness.[51] It is perhaps no surprise that the Abbé Grégoire coined the neologism *vandalism* two months later.[52]

Radical Revolutionary Cemeteries

In addition to destroying the remains of France's dead elite, radical revolutionaries during the Terror also attempted to create new, highly politicized spaces for the ordinary dead. Most famously, in the autumn of 1793—concurrent with the Saint-Denis exhumations—Joseph Fouché and Anaxagoras (né Pierre-Gaspard) Chaumette took concrete steps to secularize and radicalize cemeteries in Paris and beyond. Fouché would eventually become Napoleon's infamous head of police, but in late 1793 he was an elected representative in the National Convention, on mission in France's center and counterrevolutionary west. Chaumette was the ultraradical *procureur syndic* (an elected, executive-level magistrate) of the Paris Commune during the Terror. Chaumette and Fouché are two of the best-known revolutionaries associated with the phenomenon that is generally referred to as "de-Christianization"—an iconoclastic movement in October and November 1793 in which particularly zealous republicans attempted to excise all aspects of Christianity from French public life.[53] On October 10, 1793, Fouché passed a law in the city of Nevers in the center of France that outlined a new religious policy for a nation that recognized no cult or dogma other than that of "universal morality." Fouché's decree is so well known among historians of the Revolution that it has become a metonym for de-Christianization.[54] The care and administration of the dead was central to the decree.

Three of the seven articles in Fouché's decree concerned the dead. First, he insisted that every citizen be transported to a designated municipal building twenty-four hours after death (forty-eight if their death had been sudden). They were then to be covered with a funeral shroud painted with an "image of sleep." Next, their body would be transported to the communal grave by a cortège of friends (dressed in mourning clothes), a public officer, and a military detachment. He further stipulated that the communal burial space needed to be in an isolated locale, planted with trees, and featuring a solitary statue in repose. A required sign on the entry gate would read, "Death is an eternal sleep." Finally, Fouché noted that "all those who, after death, are judged by the citizens of their commune to have been worthy of the patrie, will have a wreath of oak leaves carved of stone placed on their tombs."[55] Fouché was vague on the specifics of what this process of judgment might look like.

Chaumette—a native of the Nièvre department where Nevers was located—was present when Fouché passed his decree. Although historians have disagreed over the relative influence that these men had over one another and their role in the genesis of de-Christianization, it will suffice to state that both were active, eager, and effective agents for a wholly secular republic.[56] Several days after Fouché issued his decree, Chaumette promoted it at the general council meeting of the Paris Commune. Two days after that, on October 18, he suggested similar reforms for the capital. Specifically he insisted that all Parisians, regardless of wealth, be afforded the same honors after death; he charged the police with providing coffins for those who could not afford them (the cost would be offset by the higher fees that the wealthy would pay).[57] A month later, Chaumette called on city administrators to enact even more radical measures, which were nearly identical to Fouché's October decree. This included a cemetery sign announcing that "the just man never dies, he lives in the memory of his fellow citizens" and a tricolored mortuary sheet to be draped over the coffins of the dead, as a symbol of patriotism and political unity.[58]

These radical plans met with limited success. While superficial reforms were implemented in Paris and Nevers, they quickly became unpopular and controversial. Several months after the height of the de-Christianization frenzy of autumn 1793, both Fouché and Chaumette ran afoul of Robespierre and his ruling coterie in the Committee of Public Safety. Chaumette went the guillotine with the extreme-left, so-called "Hébertistes" in April 1794. When Robespierre attempted to similarly expel Fouché from the Jacobin club in July, it ultimately motivated Fouché to conspire with other revolutionaries to orchestrate Robespierre's downfall. In his final speech to the National Convention, just hours before his arrest and execution, Robespierre reiterated his opposition to the October 10 decree, announcing, "No, Fouché, death is not an eternal sleep. Citizens, wipe from the tombs this impious phrase which throws a funeral shroud over nature and insults the dead! Write in its place this: death is the beginning of immortality!"[59] As reviled as Robespierre became after his death, his critique of these aggressively secular cemeteries took root and blossomed in the years after the Terror. As late as 1796, Parisians were openly complaining about the silliness of draping a tricolor sheet over every casket.[60] And, as future chapters will elaborate, the bogeyman of the atheistic revolutionary cemetery was a powerful trope in appeals for urban burial reform for at least a decade after 1794.

Fouché and Chaumette garner a great deal of attention from historians because of their radicalism. But their policies—while extreme—were largely superficial transformations of existing burial spaces; neither man attempted to craft legislation that would comprehensively overhaul French burial culture. Other, less flashy revolutionaries were thinking about broader reforms that could be enacted on a nationwide scale. For example, Jean-Charles Leveaux, editor of the radical newspaper *Journal de la montagne*, published a lengthy editorial outlining his suggestions for reform. When discussing the illustrious dead, Leveaux's ideas closely resembled what the architect Vaudoyer had proposed in 1791: he suggested burying the nation's great men in an accessible outdoor venue, such as the Champ de Mars. However, Leveaux was not content with a plan that was limited to France's few elite heroes. He also envisioned a new commemorative culture for ordinary French citizens that would foster patriotic sentiment and social cohesion, but without all the mess of cemeteries. Instead, he imagined a scenario in which citizens would bury their loved ones in their own private gardens. These small pieces of the patrie would be "sacred" to the families and would fulfill multiple purposes for the fledgling republic. In addition to providing a diffuse solution to the burial crisis, these miniature garden cemeteries would be the perfect venue for any ceremonies or contracts in which individuals wished to engage. As Leveaux explained, who would dare violate an oath sworn over the bones of their dead ancestors? Moreover, these garden graves would help maintain the unity and indivisibility of the nation by keeping the population in place. Again, who would voluntarily sell or abandon the land that harbored their relatives? This kind of anchoring device was particularly valuable in 1793, when emigration from France had reached record highs.[61]

Leveaux's innovative scheme also highlights a significant shift that was taking place in attitudes about the relationship between emulation, commemoration, and the dead. If the Panthéon exemplified a revolutionary valorization of "great men," then Leveaux's garden cemeteries presented this phenomenon in a democratized (and domesticated) form.

This phenomenon is inseparable from the eighteenth-century concept of emulation, which John Shovlin concisely defined as "a form of gentlemanly competitiveness" and "a drive to imitate or surpass others in virtue and merit."[62] Conventionally, emulation referred to a desire to replicate the inspiring examples of ancient heroes, whether through exemplary acts of bravery or erudition. However, as many scholars have demonstrated, emulation underwent significant changes over the course of the eighteenth century. Most notably, as the century sped toward revolution, Enlightenment authors increasingly invested emulation with the power to construct civic virtue and shape social behavior.[63] By 1793, when Leveaux, Chaumette, and Fouché were writing about burial reform, emulation had become central to the republican educational project of civic regeneration. In clubs, festivals, and the public sessions of the National Convention, patriotic and virtuous citizens were routinely celebrated and rewarded for acts worthy of widespread emulation.[64] The dead certainly appeared in many of these celebrations, whether as individuals whose lives had been worthy of emulation, such as Mirabeau, or those whose deaths elevated them to greatness, including "martyrs" like Marat, Bara, and Viala. However, revolutionary writings on burial reform radically widened the scope of emulation. The dead could inspire not only through exemplary feats of courage and patriotism, but also through consistent daily acts of private virtue.

Early in 1794, the Parisian Department of Public Works crafted its own plan for burial reform, which reflected this expanded notion of emulation. An administrator in that department, Jean-Baptiste Avril, first delivered a detailed report to the general council of the Paris Commune on January 10.[65] Obviously, Avril noted, the department would take measures to ensure that it protected public health at all costs, but this was not the dominant theme of the report. Instead, it focused on the myriad ways that new cemeteries could be integrated into republican culture and used in such a way to foster greater social cohesion, political virtue, and patriotic devotion among the population. Significantly, Avril and his colleagues firmly believed that as a moment of extreme regeneration and rebirth, the Revolution presented the perfect opportunity to reconsider the instructional potential of a properly conceived civic burial culture.

In his lengthy report, Avril detailed the physical features of the Department of Public Works' proposed new burial spaces. Like many before (and after) him, Avril proposed four "fields of rest" (*champs de repos*) for large urban areas like Paris—one for each corner of the city—of approximately one square kilometer (twenty arpents) each. Avril also eschewed the Old Regime aesthetic of memento mori or any macabre imagery like skulls and skeletons. Instead, each cemetery would feature a variety of trees, green grasses, and fragrant flowers to please, rather than frighten visitors. Aside from landscape architecture, the proposed décor was sparse: in lieu of individual tombstones, a series of tablets would stand throughout the cemetery, each dedicated to a different virtue, such as filial piety, generosity, and patriotism. Citizens who exemplified these virtues would have their names inscribed on the appropriate tablet after their death. The only other monument would be in the very center of the field, which was to feature an inspiring—if someone convoluted—allegorical monument. Avril described his vision of a statue representing the earth wrapped in a cloak with the withered limbs of an old man peeking out. On one side of the man lay a cornucopia with a suckling child emerging from it, who, with one hand extended, presented the goddess Minerva to any spectators. The base of the monument featured a simple inscription reminding visitors that "virtue survives."[66]

Underpinning all of these practical details was the basic principle that Paris's new cemeteries needed to both honor the dead and contribute to the regeneration of a more virtuous population. For the dead, the proposed cemetery offered an unprecedented measure of respect and equality. Avril explained how in the future these cemeteries would significantly change the way individuals were buried: instead of packing hundreds of bodies into deep open mass graves, dead Parisians would be buried in a single layer, covered by only two feet of earth. This unconventional horizontal burial would have the double benefit of hastening decomposition and providing a pleasing analog of political equality. The proscription of tombstones, mausoleums, or any other individual monuments further guaranteed that poverty would never be a barrier to a decent burial. Far from being a marker of one's social standing, a place in the Parisian cemetery of the future was a just reward for those who had dedicated themselves to the nation, and to their fellow citizens.

In addition to attending to the needs of the dead, Avril's new fields of rest would also benefit the living. As the cemeteries' design and appearance made clear, these were places that invited, anticipated, and encouraged living guests. Although they would be walled for security reasons, these spaces would theoretically function as what one scholar has called "welcome centers" (*centres d'acceuil*) for the living.[67] Beyond merely welcoming the living, however, Avril explained that he fully expected his field of rest to "sow the seeds of heroic and social virtues" among those who passed through its gates, including "the wife who comes to mourn her husband, the son who asks for his father back, and the tearful friend." For each of these prospective visitors, the cemetery was designed to nourish a sense of loss while inspiring them to become better citizens. The careful management and organization of space was essential for the didactic potential of cemeteries to flourish. As Avril asked his audience of Parisian administrators: "Citizens, do you want to instruct usefully? Then speak to the eyes to alight the spirit and inspire the soul."[68]

Although the local government responded quite favorably to Avril's reform plan, it ultimately failed. The closest it came to fruition may have been in March 1794, when a deputation from the Paris Commune requested that the National Convention authorize them to purchase four kilometers of land on the city's periphery to provide space for the city's new cemeteries.[69] The convention referred them to the Committee of Public Instruction and nothing developed further. Two years later the Avril report was resubmitted to the minister of the interior, on the grounds that since the plan was only promulgated at the height of the Terror, "the events that followed did not permit us to follow through with its execution."[70] Although Avril's plan differed quite significantly from Fouché and Chaumette's de-Christianized spaces of death, it would never be able to rid itself of the stigma of atheism that characterized the most high-profile conversations about burial reform during the Terror.

Meanwhile, in Lyon . . .

In March 1789, just weeks before the Estates General met, a Lyonnais physician named Jean-Jacques Coindre presented a plan for burial reform to his city's municipal government. His concerns were typical of the late Old Regime. In particular, he emphasized the utmost necessity of relocating burial spaces from the interior of cities to the periphery. Coindre outlined the scourge of decomposing bodies, whose pestilential vapors he blamed for a constant stream of urban illnesses and deaths. He strongly suggested that Lyon could address this problem quickly and efficiently by building three new suburban cemeteries. He dedicated much of his essay to precise measurements and calculations about the parameters of each cemetery, the shape and depth of each cemetery's mass graves, and the number of corpses that could be safely packed into each grave. Each cemetery was to be located far outside of city limits and surrounded by a six-foot wall that would further isolate the dead and prevent them from contaminating the community of the living. While he made certain gestures toward aesthetics and landscape architecture, Coindre premised virtually every feature of his system on the necessity of establishing clean, hygienic, and safe spaces for the dead.[71]

Five years later, in 1794, a municipal committee in Lyon proposed a similar, but much more radical plan for burial reform. Like Coindre, they suggested building on elevated terrain that had good airflow and was far from any habitation, but they focused significantly less on the logistics of burial and more on the effect that this space would have on anyone who visited it. They made no mention of the size or shape of the graves, but wistfully described all citizens mingling together in eternal repose in the communal grave. Moreover, while they recommended constructing this "final retreat" (*dernier asyle*) a safe distance away from the living population, the committee wanted it to remain visible from a great distance so that the citizens of Lyon would always be aware that they were in close proximity to generations of their ancestors. They expected that this peaceful space would immediately stimulate the senses of visitors as they thought about their dearly departed friends and family members. In the end, the committee explained, anyone who passed through these cemeteries would emerge as a better, more virtuous citizen.[72]

These Lyonnais proposals closely mirrored the shift in the Parisian attitudes about burial reform during the tumultuous first five years of the French Revolution. Between 1789 and the end of the Terror in 1794, the place and function of the cemetery in the social imagination changed dramatically: it transformed from a pestilential problem in need of repair to a potentially powerful urban space at the heart of the republican cultural project of social and moral regeneration. This was not a coincidence; the experience of the Revolution dramatically altered the terms of debate when it came to burial reform. It made spaces for the dead into essential and valuable sites for civic education. In newly designated and demarcated spaces, the dead would inspire emulation, provide a theater for enacting revolutionary values, and create an ancestral foundation rooted in the soil of the fledgling patrie. These lofty goals may have been unattainable in the short run, but by 1794 they had become fundamental to the conversation about burial reform and would have a lasting impact on the way Parisians thought about the dead and their spaces for generations.

THE SOLUTION OF THE DEAD

Despite revolutionaries' lofty goals, the actual experience of the dead in Paris by 1794 was bleak. In stark contrast to the large, green, suburban cemeteries that populated the imaginations (and pamphlets) of reform-minded Jacobins, urban burial between 1789 and 1794 was as bad—quite possibly worse—than it had been under the Old Regime. In contrast to the elaborate celebrations of illustrious dead French citizens, from Mirabeau to Marat, the ordinary dead continued to fester in small, overcrowded, ad hoc cemeteries throughout the city. In 1794 a Parisian lawyer named Gaspard Delamalle exposed the state of Parisian cemeteries for those who had not yet witnessed it for themselves. In his essay *Reflections on My Mother's Burial,* Delamalle recounted the series of indignities that his mother had endured in the days following her death. As he described it, his disappointment began even before his mother's corpse left home, when virtually no one showed up to pay their respects during a period of visitation. Delamalle and his father then accompanied municipal porters as they carried his mother's simple wooden coffin to the local cemetery, the Cimetière de la barrière blanche near Montmartre. En route they encountered several unsavory characters who hollered at them, stumbled absentmindedly into the coffin, and engaged the porters in casual conversation. When the small cortège finally arrived at its final destination, Delamalle had a difficult time distinguishing the cemetery from its surroundings because nothing obvious announced that they were in a sacred place of burial; there were no signs, banners, or monuments in sight. On closer inspection he perceived a nearly unnavigable muddy path leading the way to a heaping pile of earth and rubble in the distance. "The appearance of this depot of the dead revolted me," he explained, because it "offered nothing but a spectacle of filth." Delamalle and his father made their way through the muck, almost falling several times, until they finally arrived at a gaping communal grave that exuded a distinctive "cadaverous odor." Delamalle recoiled at the knowledge that by sundown his dear mother's corpse would be mingling with the rest of the rotting cadavers in the "cesspool called a grave" before him. He returned home, full of sorrow for his lost mother but also ashamed to live in a society that virtually abandoned its citizens after death.[1]

Delamalle's critique initially seems like a return to prerevolutionary concerns about salubrity, but it actually reveals a qualitative shift. Five years of intense politicization had altered the Parisian public's understanding of the role of the dead in their city. By the end of the Terror, spaces for the dead were inextricably linked to the republican project of moral and civic regeneration. The inability of the new state to care for its citizens after their death was more than a public health crisis, it also reflected a crisis of moral health after the Terror. As Delamalle asked, immediately after painting this grim portrait of his mother's burial: "Did we think that ceremonies and funeral monuments were contrary to equality and Republican simplicity? It is in Republics above all that such institutions are necessary: There can be no Republic without *moeurs*."[2] Delamalle's castigation of his city's burial practices reveals the gaping void that existed between revolutionary ideals and their application by the end of the Terror. Delamalle was particularly vexed by the degraded and degrading application of "equality" in the cemetery, which exposed all corpses to the same indignities. He wholeheartedly agreed with the basic principle of providing every citizen with the same treatment after death, but emphasized how badly the revolutionaries had missed their mark. These shortcomings of the Revolution are well-trod territory among historians, particularly among those who have examined the revolutionaries' unsuccessful attempts to supplant Catholic with secular republican traditions.[3] However, while these large-scale projects often backfired in the short term, they did not simply fade away into obscurity. Rather, as this chapter demonstrates, the failure of some of the Revolution's first round of civic reforms actually gave new energy to those interested in continuing this difficult work after 1794.

While Delamalle mercilessly criticized the funerary and burial practices of his day, he also put forward a very clear articulation of why reform was necessary for the future success of the republic. "Care of funerals and tombs honors divinity, humanity, society, [and] virtue," he explained. "It nourishes all the noble sentiments of the heart, it inspires respect for filial piety, it places value on domestic virtues, and it inspires all good citizens to do well by their patrie."[4] Delamalle's essay was more than a scathing exposé; it was also a call to action and a reaffirmation of the cohesive and socially constructive power of a well-ordered cemetery.

Critiques like Delamalle's revealed deep anxieties about the corrosive social effects of the Revolution, which many Parisians, from neighborhood groups to elected officials, began expressing in the aftermath of the Terror. Not only were disheveled burial sites evidence of revolutionary mismanagement, they were increasingly interpreted as signs of a deeper crisis of social and moral disorder in the capital. Parisians were concerned about their shabby cemeteries in part because they worried that basic human social practices—such as properly burying the dead—had been lost in the revolutionary haste to demolish, innovate, and re-create France anew. However, as the previous chapter demonstrated the Revolution also opened up wide new avenues of possibility for the dead as a constructive and stabilizing force in the city. By the end of the eighteenth century, reformers dreamed up a range of mechanisms by which carefully designed cemeteries would avert and resolve what they perceived as a looming crisis of social disorder. They stretched the limits of their imaginations and designed new didactic spaces for the dead that included instructions for turning bones into glass, procedures for holding postmortem trials, and designs for double cemeteries that separated virtuous from reprobate citizens. The authors of these projects intended to do significantly more than improve burial practices; they hoped that their new cemeteries would complete the work of the Revolution by restoring social order, morality, and civic responsibility among a population they thought had been badly— but not irreparably—damaged by the experience of the previous decade.

Depots for the Dead

When the Cemetery of the Innocents closed in 1780, prerevolutionary re- formers had high hopes for a new and improved set of burial practices in the capital. Revolutionaries like Jean-Baptiste Avril eagerly took up this mantle, but tailored it to suit republican ideals. However, as Gaspard Delamalle's essay makes clear, these lofty goals ultimately sank in the mire of temporary, ad hoc graveyards throughout the city. As many had done before the Revolution, city dwellers after the end of the Terror regu- larly petitioned the municipal and national authorities to have their neigh- borhood cemeteries closed down. Their complaints usually reached fever pitch during the summer months, when the extreme heat exacerbated the smell emanating out of the "graves of putrefaction" and allegedly made daily life unbearable for individuals who lived nearby.[5] However, the ex- perience of the Revolution, and the Terror in particular, added a new dimension to these complaints: the only thing worse than a pile of decom- posing bodies in the middle of one's neighborhood was a pile of decom- posing bodies without their heads.

One of the most notorious cemeteries of the Terror opened suddenly in summer of 1794 in the courtyard of a former convent on the south- eastern edge of the city.[6] Although this cemetery, known as Picpus, has since become famous as the posh private cemetery where the Marquis de Lafayette is buried, the revolutionary state initially established it to con- tain the bodies of individuals who had just been executed at the nearby Barrière du trône renversé (present-day Place de la Nation).[7] After only a few weeks of operation, local residents began complaining about the presence of so many decapitated corpses in their neighborhood. As one complainant noted, three hundred republican students and countless el- derly French citizens were "justifiably alarmed" by their proximity to this new space, whose sole purpose was to contain "conspirators struck down by the sword of justice."[8] One individual, Antoine Riédain, was especially indignant. He was the primary occupant of the adjacent building and had been leasing the property from the state for months. Riédain also made his living off of the property by subleasing a large part of the building to a local entrepreneur. As he described it, in the spring of 1794—the height of the Terror—a small group representing the Department of Public Works showed up to tour the property. He claimed to have thought nothing much of the visit and was shocked when, on June 13, the same department dispatched a group of laborers to smash a hole in his garden wall and begin digging a deep mass grave to accommodate the decapitated victims of the guillotine. When Riédain protested, none other than Jean-Baptiste Avril informed the angry resident that the national good took precedence over the individual good and there was nothing he could do to prevent the establishment of a cemetery for counterrevolutionaries in his courtyard. For the next two months, Riédain had the displeasure of watching city workers bury almost fifteen hundred decapitated bodies in large open graves just outside of his windows, allegedly at all hours of the day and night. He claimed that his spouse had become "sick from horror and fright" from the "unhappy operation" and had to relocate to a different apartment across town for four months.[9] Although the mass burials only lasted until the end of the Terror in August, the grave remained open for another year. Riédain believed that these months of suffering entitled him to an indemnity of twenty-four hundred francs, which the state eventually awarded him. As an architect for the Department of Public Works noted after reviewing Riédain's case a year later, "The frightening service that citizen Riédain was subjected to, of being the daily witness to a repulsive spectacle" certainly justified his request for compensation.[10] Ironically, while revolutionaries had energetically banished Catholic memento mori from their cemeteries, they ultimately created a new breed of urban burial space that was significantly more terrifying to contemporaries than a skull and crossbones.

Like his contemporary Gaspard Delamalle, Riédain lodged his complaint during a particularly fraught political climate, generally known as the Thermidorian period: a thirteen-month interval between the end of the Terror and the beginning of a new moderate republican government. As many historians have argued, this interregnum was a time of reaction, uncertainty, and confusion as revolutionaries struggled to condemn the violence of the Terror without losing sight of the republican project to create a more just and equitable social order, free from the corrupting influence of the monarchy and church.[11] Critiques of Paris's burial culture latched on to the prevailing narrative of urgency. In April 1795 the *Moniteur universel* published a letter by Charles-Joseph Trouvé about the treatment of the dead in Paris in which Trouvé commended Delamalle's essay and urged the National Convention to address the city's cemetery crisis as soon as possible. This kind of immediate reform, he explained, would not only help the Thermidorians separate themselves from the government of the Terror, it would begin the much-needed process of restoring stability in the French capital. Trouvé emphasized that rituals and spaces for the dead were absolutely essential institutions that would preserve society by fostering and maintaining public and private virtue among the population.[12]

By September 1795, France had a new constitution and a moderate republican government known as the Directory, so called for its five-man executive committee that went by the same name. This regime was long infamous for its corruption, inefficiency, and instability, although scholars have recently reinterpreted this maligned era as a time when republicans consolidated key elements of modern French civic culture.[13] This was also a period when the state energetically took up the project of cemetery reform and set the stage for the comprehensive legislation and construction projects of the Napoleonic Era. As early as October 1795, the Department of Public Works embarked on a thorough survey of Parisian cemeteries and their environs. The resulting report observed that despite existing laws that prohibited urban interment, only two of Paris's seventeen cemeteries were actually located outside of the city's walls. Moreover, the contemporary method of burial—of tightly packing bodies into deep holes in the ground—was impractical, insalubrious, and insupportable. The report strongly advised that the state return to Jean-Baptiste Avril's 1794 plan to establish four suburban cemeteries that used long shallow trenches as mass graves, instead of deep pits. It also recommended against the use of porters and suggested that that horse-drawn carts would be a more efficient method of transporting the dead to cemeteries. Most significantly, the Department of Public Works recommended closing all but five of the city's active cemeteries.[14]

When the state took up the Department of Public Works's recommendation and reduced the number of Parisian burial spaces by more than half, it placed an immediate burden on the remaining five. For individuals who lived in close proximity to these sites, the influx of new bodies was unacceptable. Throughout the summer and fall of 1796, residents and officials from Paris's first arrondissement repeatedly implored the minister of the interior to close down their local cemetery, Errancis (adjacent to Parc Monceau and often referred to as the Monceau cemetery), which quickly became an overflowing "foyer de corruption."[15] These petitions contained both familiar and innovative arguments, revealing the subtle but significant shift in the public's perception of their cemeteries after the Terror. According to letters and petitions sent to the minister of the interior, mephitic vapors were seeping out of overflowing mass graves and killing off local animals—complaints that Parisians had been making against their urban cemeteries for decades. Yet, interspersed among arguments about hygiene and public health were distinctly political claims that reflected the reactionary fervor of the time. Petitioners who lived near Monceau repeatedly invoked the fact that their cemetery had violent origins, explaining that it was only during the Terror that the followers of Robespierre had "revolutionarily seized" a portion of their park because they needed a place to stash their decapitated victims.[16] They claimed that as of 1796 their cemetery contained upwards of four thousand of these "victims of the terrorists."[17] In the wake of the Terror, the city's existing cemeteries had become more than a threat to public health, they were also disquieting reminders of recent violence, disorder, and uncertainty.

Concerned observers also linked Parisian cemeteries to the Terror is less direct ways. They pointed to disturbingly antisocial behavior among the population, similar to what Delamalle recorded, and interpreted it as an unfortunate consequence of revolutionary upheaval and dislocation. Jean-Marie Coupé, a former Jacobin and elected representative to the Directory's lower house, the Council of Five Hundred, first addressed Paris's cemetery crisis in the summer of 1796, spelling out the deplorable "apathy of our era" in which he regularly encountered coffins laying in the middle of the street, and where the city's cemeteries bore the "hideous and barbaric" appearance of charnel houses.[18] That same summer, Emmanuel Pastoret lamented that since the Revolution began, "brutal men" had been unleashing their "sacrilegious vengeance" on the dead by violating tombs and playing with human bones.[19] Two years later, Jean-Marie Lafargue described Parisian cemeteries as spaces of "anarchy" and disorder. In his analysis, the situation had deteriorated to such an extreme that barely buried cadavers were becoming playthings for wild animals. "If one must provoke horror to motivate urgency," he exclaimed, "I will tell you that I witnessed a tearful mother fighting with a wild pig over the cadaver of her beloved child."[20] Using similarly evocative language, Marie-Nicolas-Sylvestre Guillon, a priest, ended the eighteenth century with a brutal description of contemporary Paris: "Only the genius of destruction remains standing in this bloody ocean that surrounds us," he wrote. "Everything has been turned upside down and mixed together. Mutilated limbs lay everywhere, disgusting tatters; scattered and broken bones; the cadaver of a stranger lays next to my father's as though on a battlefield."[21] By the end of the century, cemeteries had become a kind of barometer for the social and political uncertainty that Parisians witnessed all around them.

Grave robbing, lazy porters, and disorderly cemeteries were familiar problems in Paris, but critics after the Terror addressed them in a new way. For them, this was more than a logistical problem or a public safety concern; it revealed a deeper and more pernicious crisis of moral health. Virtually everyone who wrote about burial reform during this time, from devout Catholics to former Jacobin radicals, agreed that commemorating the dead was a basic human impulse. As Arsenne Thiébault, a young soldier and intellectual, and put it: "This sentiment, this respect for death is engraved on our souls: the wildest man shares this with the man of order; it has been consecrated at all times and in all places."[22] That Parisians were unwilling or unable to honor their dead was widely interpreted as disturbingly unnatural. The celebrated poet Gabriel Legouvé implored his reader in *La Sépulture:* "And you, polite people, in this beautiful age, where Montesquieu, Voltaire, Raynal and Rousseau taught the dignity of man through their brilliant writings, you alone dare to refuse to honor the dead!"[23] France, it seemed, was betraying not only nature but also its own character with its poor treatment of the dead.

The Rebirth of Burial Reform

After five years of chaos-laden criticism regarding burial practices, the idea of reform finally revived in 1799. Several weeks after Napoleon Bonaparte seized power in November 1799, the Department of the Seine approved and widely distributed a new report about the city's cemeteries by the former administrator Jacques Cambry. Cambry announced that of all the populations in history, contemporary Parisians were the most cruel and least respectful toward their dead, but he saw potential in the chaos that surrounded him. As he encouraged Parisian administrators: "You want to do good; you are working to repair the harm and disturbances (*désordres*) that are inseparable from such a massive revolution." He then promised them that it was very possible to restore order, nature, sensibility, and the much-needed "religion of tombs" in the French capital.[24] Just as spaces and rituals associated with the dead could be used to diagnose a badly damaged population, reforming and rebuilding them would ultimately regenerate that same population. This argument was very much in line with the thinking of its time. Bonaparte vigorously continued the Directory's goal of building a firm institutional foundation for France. Scholars usually point to Napoleon's "blocks of granite" as evidence of this restabilization—higher education, the military, and a comprehensive legal code—but Bonaparte also recognized the pressing need for burial reform.[25]

In 1800 Napoleon's younger brother Lucien, who was then the minister of the interior, inspired an unprecedented number of cemetery reform projects. He instructed the French National Institute to issue an essay-writing contest on the subject of suitable regulations for burial and funerals.[26] At the time, the institute had only been in operation for five years, but it replaced the much older French Academy, which dated back to 1634. The academy had begun with a mandate to conserve and regulate the French language, but by the second half of the eighteenth century it had begun to address issues such as political liberty and social equality. This new emphasis was reflected in the academy's tradition of sponsoring prize contests. Most famously, Jean-Jacques Rousseau's *Discourse on Inequality* had been a response to a contest from the Academy of Dijon and Robespierre's treatise against the death penalty won first prize in a competition from the Academy of Metz. Despite these close ties with the Enlightenment, radical revolutionaries shut down all of France's academies in the summer of 1793.

Two years later, the same constitution of 1795 that established the Directory also reestablished the academies under the new name National Institute and charged it with "the collection of discoveries, with the improvement of the arts and the sciences."[27] The institute almost immediately resumed the prize competitions, issuing at least one per year. The 1800 competition addressing burial reform was by far the most popular and successful. The competition was open to the public and asked respondents to answer two questions: "What kind of ceremonies should one have for funerals?" and "What regulations should be adopted for places of burial?" It received forty complete entries—significantly more than any of the institute's other contests on moral or political topics. Submissions came from all over France and from a range of professional men, from farmers, to mathematicians, to previously noble men of letters. Interested individuals continued to send unsolicited proposals for cemetery reform to the Ministry of the Interior, but after 1800 they were all redirected to the institute's competition.[28] By the turn of the century, the nation's political and intellectual elites were taking very seriously the problem of the dead.

Underpinning the institute's essay question (and the responses it received) was an assumption that there was an inherent connection between death rituals and moeurs—the cultural habits, customs, and behavior of the population. The official French dictionary from 1798 defined *moeurs* as "natural or acquired habits, for good or bad, in everything that concerns the conduct of life."[29] English-speaking historians of this period have thoughtfully interpreted the term to mean both "social morals" and "culture."[30] Fréderick Mollès, a participant in the institute competition, best explained this relationship when he wrote: "If anything can restore man's good *moeurs* and social virtues, it is assuredly the view of a coffin and a grave. One often sees a villain laughing at the sight of a prepared scaffold," he noted "but rarely at the sight of a dead man whose pale and livid face is contorted with the signs of pain or despair."[31]

When authors referenced moeurs in this way they tapped into a decades-old conversation whereby sociability was a real and viable alternative to traditional sources of moral and social authority, such as the Catholic Church, the monarchy, and the hierarchy of corporate society. Like Enlightenment authors before them, these cemetery reformers argued that compassion, respect for nature, and a strong sense of patriotism would provide the social glue necessary to hold Paris (and France) together after the cataclysm of Revolution. Spaces and rituals associated with the dead were at the heart of this process. Jean-Marie Coupé invoked all of this in his 1796 essay about the politics and morals of burial practices. Death, he maintained, had both natural and moral characteristics. As a natural phenomenon, death was "a necessary end, an unfeeling sleep" in which the body returned to the earth and organic matter transformed into something new. From a moral perspective, however, death was "a supreme power" that had the possibility to influence and direct social behavior.[32] For Coupé, the pain and suffering that naturally occurred at the grave of a loved one was a powerful bond that could be used to hold society together.[33] One of Coupé's peers similarly referred to burial as the final moment of contact between the living and the dead when "all the pores of sentiment" opened wide.[34] To both men, it was essential, moral, and just for the state to take advantage of the socially cohesive properties of spaces and rituals associated with the dead.

Exploiting death in this way was nothing new. As many authors eagerly pointed out, the Catholic Church had been doing it for generations, but they had used this power for self-interest rather than the good of the community. In his contest essay a lawyer from Champagne, Thomas Doderet, argued that during the Old Regime priests had converted cemeteries into veritable gold mines.[35] François René Jean de Pommereul, a military general, similarly decried the Catholic Church as an "exclusive and dominating cult" that had taken advantage of funerals and death rituals for financial gain. Indeed, Pommereul (rather uniquely) blamed the Old Regime rather than the Revolution for the sorry state of France's burial culture in the 1790s. "It is not because the nation lost its sensibility" he explained, "but solely because all of the exterior funeral rites belonged to a privileged cult that usurped the right to have, and direct funerals."[36] This hostility toward the Old Regime is surprising since Pommereul had every reason to be resentful toward the radical revolutionaries: his wife and children had been imprisoned in Paris during the Terror while he was denied permission to reenter France from Italy on the grounds that he had emigrated while serving in the military. With only slightly less invective, an artist and musician named Pagès, noted that while burial was "a sacred duty that nature has imposed on man since the beginning of time" it was a duty that religious leaders had previously exploited for their own gain. "Today," he explained "society, enlightened about all pointless superstitions, must reclaim its rights."[37]

General hostility toward the corruption of the Catholic Church was matched by a nearly wholesale rejection of Fouché and Chaumette's infamously "de-Christianized" cemeteries of the Terror. A former judge from the Loire-Atlantique neatly captured the middle ground that so many cemetery reformers aspired to at the end of the century. He explained that he and his countrymen were "revolted" in equal measure by the Old Regime's ostentatious display of inequality and the "apathetic coldness" of the Revolution. Reflecting the spirit of the times, in which moderate republicans attempted to chart a political course between the extremes of right and left, he announced that for cemeteries, as in all things, a *juste milieu* was the answer.[38] Joseph de Girard wrote one of the most impassioned appeals for this kind of moderate middle ground. A former (and future) nobleman who was most famous for being the brother of the man who invented the flax-spinning machine, Girard entered the institute's essay competition with the goal of writing a "simple and moral" plan that would inspire tender sentiment rather than somber reflection among its readers. He took seriously the problem of religion and unpacked the complex relationship between death, cemeteries, and "superstition." Although his essay received an honorable mention rather than the grand prize, he later expanded and published his work in Paris. As one contemporary newspaper noted, Girard spared none of the shameful details of France's past and made salient observations about both the "fanaticism of superstition" and the social danger of materialism.[39]

Like many of his colleagues, Girard began his book by describing religious beliefs as disparate as ancient Greek, Christian, and Native American. His initial goal was to prove that consoling acts of mourning and narratives of eternity were a universal response to loss. However, after establishing this generally agreed-on truism, Girard extended his analysis to explain how the pernicious habit of "superstition" was itself born out of tombs. When motivated by the twin fears of death and eternal punishment, man had a tendency to abandon the "light of reason" in favor of "insane vows" which "inverted" the laws of nature. Specifically, Girard lamented the history of religious wars in which men blindly killed each other in the name of a wrathful god. Because of this potentially dangerous connection, Girard cautioned that proper death rituals were of the utmost importance for a nation in the process of redefining its religious identity. "The legislator must be vigilant" he insisted, "to push away futile terrors that enchain the imagination." Instead, "he must use funeral flames to enlighten the people, to bring philosophy into the tomb, to dissipate the useless ghosts that 'superstition' makes out of the regular procession of the dead."[40] However, Girard also warned readers and potential legislators against the equally dangerous materialism of the Terror. At least superstition brought people together, he noted, whereas materialism destroyed "all of the magic of the social order, broke the ties between leaders, citizens, and families" and ruptured "that sacred chain that extends from the heavens for the happiness of the earth."[41] To Girard, this went against the very purpose of spaces for the dead, which he considered to be one of the best ways to reconnect neglected bonds and unite the population. "Sadness and melancholy," he explained, "bring men together much more powerfully than pleasure and interest."[42]

This moderate approach to religious policy was perfectly in line with thinking at the highest level of the state after the Terror. In 1796, Pierre-Louis Roederer had read a report before the National Institute with the telling title "Funerary Institutions Suitable for a Republic that Respects All Religious Cults but Adopts None."[43] Although the Directory fell into a brief but significant anticlerical phase after 1797, by the time Napoleon Bonaparte took power this commitment to religious conciliation was official state policy. Jacques-Olivier Boudon has demonstrated, for example, that under Bonaparte, the French state adopted a dual commitment to preserving—but controlling—the power of a Catholic Church and respecting the Enlightenment commitment to religious pluralism. In practice, this meant restoring formal ties with the pope via the Concordat of 1801, but also establishing religious institutions for Protestants and Jews, which were also under state control.[44] The long-term effect of these Napoleonic religious policies set the stage for *laïcité*, but the initial impetus was to reestablish domestic stability and maintain social order. The essays about funeral reform demonstrate how intellectuals at the end of the century similarly imagined a new, postrevolutionary culture of the dead that accomplished these same didactic goals.

Judging the Dead

When Pierre Dolivier, a history teacher and former *curé rouge* from Versailles, heard about the institute's essay contest he was instantly intrigued and excited, since it directly addressed a subject that had been troubling him for quite some time.[45] For him, participating in the competition was an excellent opportunity to resuscitate the public morality that he feared had been "nearly extinguished in all hearts" by the century's end.[46] After establishing the basic tenet that funerals needed to have a religious foundation, he proposed an eclectic mix of possible practices culled from traditions throughout time and across cultures. For example, he commended the Greek tradition of having a communal meal after a funeral as well as the Roman practice of kissing the dead one last time and closing their eyelids. More unusual, however, was his excited discussion of the "sublime institution" of judging the dead, which he ascribed to ancient Egyptians.[47] Dolivier imagined a funeral where everyone familiar with the dead gathered around the corpse, which was adorned with a small crown of fragrant herbs. The crowd would then engage in a rigorous discussion of the deceased, including everything that they knew about his actions and character. If a consensus emerged that he had lived an exemplary life, a ringing bell would triumphantly announce the verdict, he would be upgraded to a crown of flowers, and receive a great funeral at the expense of the state. If found "guilty," however, he would be stripped of his funeral crown and quickly removed from the cemetery.[48]

Dolivier's proposal was certainly odd, but it was far from unique; more than a quarter of the essays written about funeral reform between 1795 and 1800 proposed some type of posthumous judgment for citizens, whether an official trial or some other institutionalized system of differentiating the good from the wicked. Similarly, during an earlier institute essay contest, which asked respondents to propose institutions suitable for founding public morality, more than half of the entries suggested an elected or appointed board of censors who would directly reward virtue and reinforce good social behavior among the population.[49] Such heavy-handed didacticism speaks volumes about the severity with which educated and politically active elites interpreted the crisis of moeurs in France after the Terror. Perhaps it also presages the statist approach that would proliferate throughout the Consulate and Empire, where intense censorship and an extensive network of spies exerted a tremendous amount of control over civic culture.

The popularity of the death tribunal among cemetery reformers also reflects the rising popularity of "Egyptomania" in Europe at the turn of the nineteenth century, but only as inspiration. While contemporary publications about Egypt and the ancient world made passing reference to the practice of judging Pharaohs after death, the cemetery reformers exploded this concept to suit their own interests. For example, one anonymous entry to the institute's competition gave several precise definitions of "bad citizens" who needed to be excised from the community after death, including he who was willfully unemployed and refused to learn a profession or trade; he who neglected his sons' education and "let his daughters live in infamy"; a gambler, drinker, or libertine; a coward who refused to defend his country in a time of war; a tax-evader; and anyone found dead "in an infamous location, or in debauchery."[50] In his competition entry Thomas Doderet provided his readers with a practical set of yes-or-no questions, whose answers would clarify the character of every deceased person. The questions were very straightforward:

> Did the deceased behave well in the view of his mother, father, and other family members?
> In the view of his spouse?
> In the view of his children?
> Was the deceased just and incapable of doing harm to other people?
> Did the deceased enjoy doing good things for others, and providing honest services?
> Was the life of the deceased free of debauchery, disorder, and excess?

Additionally, Doderet recommended that the mortuary jury discuss the deceased's most noticeable defects, vices, and virtues. He also suggested that dead bodies ought to be examined for any outward signs of vice. If the individual distinguished themselves through contributions to the arts, sciences, or public administration, this counted in their favor, as did any education that they provided for their children.[51]

Doderet organized most of his eighty-page essay around this admittedly obscure historical practice, but his thinking was neither uninformed nor easy to dismiss. The institute awarded him an honorable mention for his work and shortly before composing his competition entry, Doderet published a lengthy volume on global religions.[52] Yet, while the Egyptian Death Tribunal was an ostensibly religious institution, the criteria for evaluating the dead was almost exclusively based on democratic citizenship and civic productivity, which makes perfect sense when one considers how much value late eighteenth-century thinkers placed on death rituals as a solution to perceived social collapse after the Terror. For Doderet, it was a dangerous error to only think of funeral ceremonies as private affairs for mourning families. "Their object is more important," he insisted. "They must contribute to the amelioration of *moeurs* by rewarding the good man with praise, and by covering the perverse man with approbation." In this way, the Death Tribunal supplemented both religion and the law because it assessed and punished (or rewarded) the kind of damaging (or constructive) social behavior that might otherwise go unchecked (or unnoticed).[53]

As much as they valued obscure funeral rituals, for reformers such as Doderet and Dolivier, the postmortem trial was a ceremonial means to a much more permanent end. Both men concluded their hypothetical systems of postmortem judgment by relocating the dead to one of several possible spaces. For Dolivier, exemplary citizens were rewarded with an honored position in the municipal cemetery, while those found "guilty" ended up in a separate cemetery for reprobates. He recognized that most citizens would fall somewhere between these two extremes, so he created a third category in which good but unexceptional citizens would occupy a less honored location in the cemetery.[54] Similarly, Doderet emphasized how important it was to separate out those who had failed their postmortem trial and condemn them to a "black cemetery" where they would be buried anonymously in a mass grave.[55] Doderet considered this a "second death, a death of ignominy" that would ultimately serve as an excellent mode of social control for the living.[56] General Pommereul proposed a very similar scheme in which a Field of Honor contrasted with a Field of Oblivion. While those contained in the latter would be soon forgotten, the most deserving citizens would have their names and a description of their good deeds permanently inscribed on the walls surrounding their field. This apotheosis, he explained, "would become one of the most powerful means to encourage all socially useful virtues."[57]

Other participants in the institute competition proposed even more elaborate and innovative methods for separating the good from the wicked after death.[58] One anonymous correspondent suggested that criminals be thematically sorted into specially designated mass graves that broadcasted their misdeeds. He proposed burying convicted grave robbers under a sign that read: "Here lie those who are being punished for having disturbed the rest of their fellow men."[59] The Parisian Pierre Gilles Gaignoeux explained that separating the good from the wicked after death was essential if one wanted cemeteries to function as important social institutions. If criminals were permitted to mingle with virtuous citizens after death, Gaignoeux attested that he would no longer believe in morality, and the cemetery would backfire by proving that there were no long-term consequences for criminal or antisocial behavior. It was imperative for public morality, he explained, that criminals be buried in a separate cemetery, free of any decorations except perhaps for jagged rocks.[60] Another anonymous contest participant suggested a similarly bleak aesthetic for the criminals' grave, proposing that it be surrounded by thorny bushes or hedges that were either barren or produced only bitter fruit.[61]

The exclusion of criminals and condemned men from cemeteries is not entirely surprising; it recalled the Old Regime practice of excluding particular groups from churchyard cemeteries based on their religion, occupation, or behavior. If Protestants, actors, and those who died by suicide could not be buried in a Catholic churchyard, it was logical for criminals and moral enemies of the republic to be similarly denied access to the civic burial space. It also seems to be an expansion and reversal of the eighteenth-century cult of great men, whereby the destruction of undesirables offered a stark contrast to the secular immortality bestowed on civic heroes.[62] At a time when the social world felt unstable to many, such crystal clear lines of demarcation would ideally bind the population together by creating an explicit set of social values and norms for the community: good parents and dedicated civil servants were in; gamblers and grave robbers were out. Managing the dead in this way would (hopefully) safeguard and strengthen the community of the living. However, the emphasis on parallel cemeteries and the detail with which authors described their reprobate cemeteries indicates that there was something else in play: in addition to sorting and evaluating the dead, cemetery reformers at the turn of the nineteenth century were very concerned about carefully manipulating and organizing the space that Paris's dead would occupy.

Gravesite Reunions

During the Revolution, cemeteries became extremely important "symbolic space," as architectural historian Richard Etlin describes it.[63] Although some authors paid a great deal of attention to issues of landscaping, signage, and other important aesthetic features in their hypothetical cemeteries, one of the most pressing and fraught discussions about cemetery space concerned the transition from communal to individual burial sites. As Jean-Baptiste Avril's 1793 report had already established, the republican approach to civic burial was based on the fundamental principle of equality. Although Avril's proposed cemetery had preserved the use of communal graves, for symbolic political reasons he was explicit about the importance of providing each individual with enough space in the grave: in his cemetery, the dead did not accumulate into haphazard piles but lay side by side as (semianonymous) individuals forming a collective whole. Similarly, while many reformers lobbied for anonymous mass graves for criminals and other undesirables, they were equally adamant that everyone else deserved a designated space of their own in the cemetery. This insistence reflected concerns about the powerful role that gravesites could play for reasons that were personal, political, or more to the point, both.

Recommendations for individual rather than communal gravesites increased as the eighteenth century came to a close. Twice, in 1796 and 1801, Jean-Marie Coupé insisted that future French rituals needed to preserve and honor the naturally leveling effect of death. However, he justified this suggestion for pragmatic as well as symbolic reasons, noting that it would always be an "asset" to link the living directly to their dead ancestors.[64] François Daubermesnil made a similar request of the Council of Five Hundred in 1796, in which he emphasized the need for a uniform and egalitarian system of burial and commemoration, but returned repeatedly to a citizen's natural right to know the place where his loved one lay buried.[65] Writing in the heavy shadow of the Terror and its chaotic anonymous graves, Daubermesnil argued that this was more than a sacred duty, it was an urgent political move. Not only would identifying the dead help the republican state distance itself from the disorder and destruction of the Terror, it would also provide a much-needed measure of stability by creating a powerful emotional bond between the citizen, the dead, and the nation. Daubermesnil clearly explained that if a citizen knew where the object of his affection lay buried, he would develop a much deeper commitment to his patrie, which he would begin to equate with "the mother who nourished him, and at whose breast he once rested." Daubermesnil hoped that this mourning citizen would become like the native inhabitants

North America, who had famously refused to comply with colonial orders to relocate their communities because they could not bear to leave their (buried) ancestors behind. Similarly, French love for the "native soil" would grow stronger and more powerful if citizens knew that it contained their forefathers.[66]

This same sentiment that linked private emotion, public space, and patriotism also appeared in the institute competition essays five years later. In the essay that shared the institute competition prize, François-Valentin Mulot made a strong case for individual gravesites as powerful links that united generations across boundaries of death and time. Mulot surmised that if his wife were to die before him, he would have an irrepressible need to regularly visit her grave and remember their life together. He hoped to eventually join her in the same tomb. He imagined a distant future in which his descendants would carefully maintain a lush garden over his grave, contemplate his life and example, and ultimately choose to be buried nearby.[67] This sentimental fantasy evoked a famous passage by the writer Bernardin de Saint-Pierre, who described the tomb as standing on the border between two worlds—a powerful liminal space where seemingly impossible reunions took place. Joseph de Girard adopted a similarly sentimental tone when discussing romantic and filial love in the cemetery: he proposed conjoined tombstones for married couples that would feature a sculpture or image of clasped hands, "the touching symbol of a union that not even death can dissolve!"[68] These examples seem to provide evidence in support of Philippe Ariès's classic claim that shifting attitudes toward death during this time reflected the growing power of private life and the bourgeois family, but as many other essays reveal, in the (hypothetical) post-Terror cemetery, the personal was intimately tied up with the political and the grave bound together more than just distant family members.

Pierre Dolivier in particular made one of the most impassioned cases for identifiable burial sites for personal as well as political reasons. Beginning on the first page of his published "Essai sur les funérailles," Dolivier drew from his own experience of burying his five-year-old son in the wake of the Terror. Without identifying the cemetery by name, Dolivier implied that it was one of the infamous mass graves that characterized Paris in the 1790s. In addition to suffering the loss of his child, Dolivier had to endure the second trauma of losing track of the boy's remains in the vast expanse of a communal grave. "If only I knew where [your remains] were located!" he lamented. "If only I could visit you from time to time and offer the tribute of my wishes and pain! If I could nourish within myself the gentle hope that I might one day mix my bones with yours!"[69] Dolivier then extrapolated from his own miserable experience of losing his young son to conclude that "a people who is without tombs and without temples, will also be without a *patrie*" because without cemeteries, a population could not feel any true connection to their homeland. "The love of one's country is always fused to the religion of tombs," he asserted, boldly concluding that without it, "love of one's country will never arise."[70]

This argument about the tight rapport between commemoration and patriotism aligned with an Enlightenment and revolutionary political culture that placed such high value on the cult of great men, whether as an impromptu cult of Jean-Paul Marat or something more institutionalized, such as the Panthéon. However, in the aftermath of the Terror, when the degrading anonymity of Parisian burial spaces had become such a reviled symbol of revolutionary failure, it had become necessary to recognize—by name and place—the ordinary as well as the exceptional after death. This lofty goal democratized an otherwise elite practice by creating a cult of *all* citizens after death, but it also (re)presented old problems in a new form. Authors like Dolivier, Girard, and Mulot all imagined their family burial plots continuing in perpetuity and acting as a powerful bridge uniting the past, present, and future. However, as they well knew, no cemetery could actually be large enough to accomplish this in the long term: the eighteenth century had repeatedly demonstrated the sobering fact that all cemeteries eventually reach capacity. This highlighted a tension at the heart of the cemetery reform movement, which pitted a desire to commemorate each individual after death against the revolutionary goal of building burial sites that treated each individual the same after death. This tension would not be resolved for another few years, when Père Lachaise Cemetery opened its gates, but it lurked in the background of some of the most inventive turn-of-the-century reform proposals.

Beyond Burial: Pierre Giraud's Solution

One of the most technically specific, if unusual, concepts for Parisian burial reform came from Pierre Giraud, a successful architect in Paris who had previously worked on the Louvre, the Hôtel national des Invalides, and the city's prisons during the Terror. Although he was temporarily unemployed in early 1794 due to a feud with one of his colleagues, Giraud managed to survive the Terror relatively unscathed and was promoted several times during the second half of the 1790s.[71] Giraud's work on prisons introduced him to many of the same problems that plagued cemetery design: both required a great deal of thought about how to manage large numbers of bodies in small spaces to avoid the spread of dangerous miasmas.[72] He first published his plan for Parisian cemeteries in 1798 and issued an expanded and updated edition in 1801.[73] Authorities never took Giraud's ideas seriously. Nevertheless, his work offers a clear—if extreme—example of how far an experienced postrevolutionary professional like Giraud could stretch the limits of his imagination when attempting to solve the complex problem of cemetery reform at the turn of the century.

Giraud envisioned a new culture of the dead in Paris that moved beyond burial. His scheme combined elements of antiquity with cutting-edge science and immediately resolved any issues related to overcrowding and public hygiene. Instead of putting their dead in the ground, Giraud proposed that the French follow in the footsteps of many ancient civilizations and institutionalize their own unique version of cremation. He described a program in which every Parisian corpse would undergo a chemical procedure that separated its flesh from its bones. Both parts would then be subjected to high temperatures that reduced flesh to ash, and converted skeletons into a hard, glassy substance, which could in turn be shaped into myriad forms. In particular, Giraud recommended that Parisians consider sculpting this "vitrified" bone into inspiring medallions that featured portraits of the dead along with inspiring epitaphs that highlighted their virtues. Their ashes could either be incorporated into the glass or in some way affixed to the back or base of the medallion. These creations would be completely miasma free and highly portable, so families could easily display them in their homes. By relocating commemoration to the home, Giraud departed significantly from both convention and many of his contemporary cemetery reformers. Although there had always been a movement in support of so-called private burial, where individuals who owned rural property could bury their loved ones on the privacy of their own land, this was never a realistic option for the vast majority of city dwellers. With his bone-medallions Giraud found a way to extend to everyone the practice of bringing the dead home.

In a list of reasons explaining why his system was perfectly suited for postrevolutionary France, Giraud invoked contemporary debates about public health, space, and moeurs. By eliminating burial altogether, Giraud solved the two most pressing problems of space and contagion, but he was equally interested in the educational potential of his plan. "Oh! How this type of monument will be useful for *moeurs*," he wrote. "How many children will be naturally deterred, in their tender youth, from a life of crime or unruliness." To further illustrate this point, Giraud described a hypothetical scenario in which an innocent young woman faced off against a vile seducer. Just as she was about to succumb to his wiles, she glanced over to a prominently displayed medallion fashioned out of her mother's vitrified bone and was instantly revived with the strength to defeat her pursuer.[74] In this melodramatic scene, the presence of the dead quite literally safeguarded the virtue of the young. Giraud was not the only one to see the potential in his proposal: when he described the vitrification process to a former administrator for the Seine Department, the administrator allegedly responded with excitement and suggested crafting a great statue of liberty out of the bones of France's fallen soldiers.[75] Just as the bones of a dearly departed mother could inspire chaste virtue in her daughter, so too could the bones of dead soldiers instill military virtue in the young men of France.

Giraud went to great lengths to make his unconventional scheme practical. The 1801 version included several scientific appendices that described precisely how to chemically separate flesh from bone and also how to turn bone into glass. But Giraud—a practicing architect—envisioned more than just a new system for handling and commemorating the dead. He also planned a large communal "champ de repos" (field of rest) for Paris, which he hoped to build adjacent to the famed Champs-Elysées (see figures 2.1 and 2.2). Giraud intended this large municipal space to host every aspect of Paris's new culture of the dead, from funerals to vitrification. He designed the champ de repos to be equal parts practical and symbolic. The periphery of the cemetery was marked out by a double-walled gallery that created an arcade decorated with antique tombs, sepulchral lamps, and hanging garlands. Columns that supported the arcade were to be constructed out of vitrified bone culled from Paris's old and condemned cemeteries. This repurposing was a pragmatic way to dispose of the problematic dead, but it also offered a powerful symbol uniting

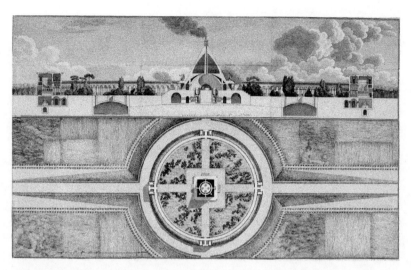

Figure 2.1. Pierre Giraud, "Cross-section of the Champ de Repos," *Les Tombeaux* (Paris, 1801). Getty Research Institute, Los Angeles (2903-530).

Paris's past with its present, whereby the city's anonymous forbears enveloped and supported its new commemorative practices. The peripheral wall featured four large pavilions, representing childhood, youth, adulthood, and old age. But the pavilions also provided lodging for cemetery employees; laboratories for doctors, surgeons, and chemists working to solve medical mysteries; and nondenominational spaces for meditation. At the center of the champ de repos stood a large pyramid topped by a blazing globe that both "neutralized putrid miasmas" and provided a beacon at night. In one of his published drawings, the pyramid exhaled plumes of smoke from several points, reminding the viewer that it was both an aesthetically pleasing focal point and a powerful furnace where all of the elaborate postmortem processes took place.[76] At every turn, the champ de repos would function efficiently for the city while also providing valuable moral instruction.

In addition to its pragmatic and moral attributes, Giraud's cemetery also contained a unique solution to the ideological problem of equality. On one hand, he applauded himself for designing a system that treated everyone the same way after death: regardless of class or religion, every person who died in Paris would enter the same pyramid and be reduced to the same skeletal contents. But Girard also recognized that the more

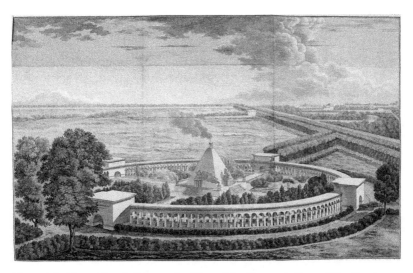

Figure 2.2. Pierre Giraud, "Perspective View of the Champ de Repos," *Les Tombeaux* (Paris, 1801). Getty Research Institute, Los Angeles (2903-530).

advanced features of his system would be out of reach for Paris's poorest citizens—he estimated the cost of the vitrification procedure at fifty francs. As an alternative to vitrification, he proposed that if these families were willing to pay a small fee to cover the cost of the (mandatory) flesh-dissolving treatment, they could recover their loved one's skeletal remains from the champ de repos and display or dispose of them in whatever manner they saw fit, provided they obtained prior permission from the state. Giraud also recognized that some skeletons might go unclaimed for any number of reasons. These abandoned bones were to be carefully labeled and stored in an underground catacomb for one year, after which point they would be vitrified, repurposed, and put into service as bricks that could be added to the columns and other structures in the champ de repos.[77] In this way, the poor would—somewhat disturbingly—retain a place in the cemetery.

Giraud's system for burial reform was exceptional in its specifics, but many of his underlying assumptions were not. The stark contrast between an individualized medallion and an anonymous brick signaled a shift in thinking about Parisian spaces for the dead at the beginning of the nineteenth century. In a widely circulated report on cemetery reform at the end of 1799, Jacques Cambry and Jacques Molinos similarly recommended radically different treatment for Paris's poor, who were to be cremated, and its wealthy, who could purchase elaborate tombs and catacombs. Cambry defended this unequal system by reminding his readers that focusing on the shape and size of a tomb was ultimately pointless: "Ah! Believe me," he explained, "death's terrifying scythe creates a level playing field that no elegant friezes, bizarre arabesques, or pompous pyramids can ever destroy."[78] Similarly, in the summer of 1800 a group of Parisian entrepreneurs proposed a tiered system of burials and commemorative monuments on the grounds that charging a high fee for lavish accommodations would make it possible to bury the poor for free.[79] That these authors, along with Giraud and Cambry felt compelled to hedge their proposals' inequality with measures (or statements) to protect the poor is telling. A new social climate was on the horizon, one that allowed for the free expression—even celebration—of socioeconomic difference in cemeteries.[80] However, in the early years of the nineteenth century, the legacy of the Revolution still loomed large, and few were willing to fully abandon equality in the treatment of the dead.

Frochot, Bonaparte, and the Imperial Decree on Burials

These complex new attitudes toward burial practices were soon reflected in laws. The first came from Paris's ambitious new prefect, Nicolas Frochot, who issued a decree on burials in March 1801. Frochot had been a close friend of Mirabeau's during the Revolution and actively participated in drafting the first French constitution. However, like many other moderate revolutionaries he fell out of favor during the Terror and lived in obscurity until Napoleon's coup d'état.[81] When Napoleon created his new administrative body, the prefectorial corps, Frochot secured the most important post as prefect of the Seine (Paris).[82] As Frochot interpreted it, prerevolutionary funerals had been horribly unjust, leaving the poor in a state of misery and abandonment, but the system of burials in the 1790s was not much better because it enveloped the rich and the poor "in the same indifference."[83] In an attempt to elevate the "decency" of burial practices, Frochot suggested several reforms aimed at ensuring a minimum standard of care for all bodies after death. He outlawed the use of common caskets, a practice in which the same wooden casket was reused for the poor. He pledged to keep burial costs as low as possible, but made provisions for the municipality to pay for the funerals of the indigent.[84] Frochot's decree guaranteed a respectable burial for the poor, but 1801 was not 1793, and Frochot made no attempt to create an egalitarian system, beyond guaranteeing a basic level of treatment for all citizens. As part of that basic treatment, he assured that everyone had the right to consecrate their loved one through the use of inscribed stones, cenotaphs, and other funeral monuments. Significantly, Frochot placed no substantial limits on what a family could do to "augment" funeral and commemoration practices using the services of private entrepreneurs.[85] Previous scholars have correctly noted that this decision to allow for ostentatious displays after death ultimately undermined the equality aspired to throughout the revolutionary period.[86] However it seems equally significant that every other feature of the 1801 law reflected years of debate, discussion, and proposals for reform.

The 1801 Parisian decree presaged Bonaparte's comprehensive "Imperial Decree on Graves [*Sépultures*]," which he issued on June 12, 1804, less than a month after the establishment of the First French Empire.[87] This was one small component of Bonaparte's broader campaign to establish domestic stability through strong institutions. The decree had five subsections and twenty-six articles. The first four sections concerned cemeteries, and reiterated many of the basic ideas that had been circulating for decades. First and foremost, no burials were permitted inside of cities or villages, and especially not in churches or other buildings of worship. Instead, special terrain, at least thirty meters outside of each city or village, would be reserved for burial. These spaces were to be organized in the safest and most hygienic way possible: they should be located on elevated terrain with northern exposure and surrounded by walls of at least two meters should surround them. Landscape architecture was highly recommended, provided the trees and plants did not interfere with the circulation of the air. The decree then supplemented these public health concerns with a discussion about the equal treatment of the dead: each burial was to take place in a separate grave, approximately two meters deep and eighty centimeters wide. A gap of thirty to forty centimeters between graves separated one from one another. Each body was to remain in its own grave for a minimum of five years. These provisions departed significantly from conventional mass graves and improved on the revolutionary plan to bury in long trenches. It reflected the thousands of pages that had been published in the previous decade that insisted on the importance of knowing the place of one's dead, if only for a few years.

However, in a move that recalled the emphasis that so many cemetery reformers placed on permanence, the Imperial Decree also created a new category of cemetery space called concessions. These could be purchased by those seeking "a distinct and separate space" of their own in the municipal cemetery. If purchased in perpetuity, these concessions could contain multiple generations in caves, monuments, mausoleums, or other tomblike structures. Curiously, however, as with so many other proposals for cemetery reform at the turn of the century, the Napoleonic decree hedged its deeply unequal system with provisions for the poor. The Imperial Decree required that in addition to paying a to-be-determined fee to their commune, those purchasing a concession would be required to make charitable donations to the poor or to hospitals, which would be supervised and authorized by the state. The fee structure for burials would all be worked out in future legislation, but the high fee that the municipality charged for elaborate funerals and concessions would ultimately offset the cost of burying the poor at the state's expense.

The Parisian cemetery culture that took shape between 1794 and 1804 bore the scars of the Terror. While anonymous mass graves had been in use for centuries—and had fallen out of favor for decades—their association with the violence, upheaval, and damage of the radical revolution made them unacceptable after 1794. As the final report for the National Institute's essay contest explained, the French had "changed and degraded so drastically" as a result of the Revolution that great action was needed in order to "resuscitate" the population.[88] New cemeteries were central to this project of regeneration, and individual gravesites were the indispensable links "at the threshold between both worlds" that brought together the dead, the living, and the postrevolutionary city. And when Paris finally built its first new cemetery on the elevated terrain east of the city known as Mont Louis, Parisians flocked to it.

3

The City of the Dead

In 1800 an anonymous author published a novella, *Le Cimetière de la Madeleine*, set in the notorious revolutionary cemetery where victims of the guillotine had been buried during the height of the Terror. It tells the story of a young man, Saint-Julien, who returned to Paris from abroad in the midst of the Terror only to be shocked and appalled by the violence and chaos that had transformed his home. Throughout the story, Saint-Julien succumbs to vengeful thoughts as he learns about the invention of the guillotine, the death of the royal couple, and the persecution of the Girondins. His longing for revenge is only quelled at the end of the story when he reunites with his long-lost love, Amélie, at her father's tomb. When Saint-Julien promises to avenge her father's death, Amélie begs him never to speak of vengeance in the hallowed grounds of a cemetery. "It is enough that hatred torments life," she explains, "it must not reach beyond the grave."[1] The novel ends several pages later, with Saint-Julien's wizened father commending the cemetery as an unexpected, but welcome, reunion site. This book took the same name of a much more popular work by J. G. Warin, but unlike Warin's virulently antirevolutionary work in which the protagonist dies on the guillotine, the anonymous author of this *Cimetière de la Madeleine* focuses on the cemetery as a site for mourning, community, and healing.[2] In the book's introduction, the author explicitly cautions his readers against the temptations of revenge, explaining that tears, not bloodshed, will ultimately heal the divisive wounds of the Revolution.[3] As Saint-Julien's father explains at the story's end, "When we cry for these august victims, there is not a family [in France] that doesn't join us."[4]

Interpreting a revolutionary cemetery as a site of reunion would have been unthinkable in 1795, but much had transpired in five years. By the beginning of the nineteenth century, cemetery reform was finally moving off of the page and into the city. The shape that Paris's new burial culture would take was certainly informed by the debates of the previous decade as well as a new conciliatory spirit of the Napoleonic era. Although *union et oubli* (unity and forgetting) would be the guiding principle of the early Restoration (c. 1814–20),[5] a different kind of *union et mémoire* proliferated in cemeteries for the entire first third of the nineteenth century when a veritable cemetery cult began to flourish.[6] This cultural moment has been well documented, but this chapter seeks to situate it within a postrevolutionary context and to demonstrate how the cemetery became a vital space for social reunion and reinvention in the wake of the Revolution.

Before visiting Paris's most famous and innovative space for the dead, Père Lachaise Cemetery, let us examine one of the city's smaller and (slightly) older sites. In the winter of 1811 Pierre-François Piétresson de Saint-Aubin visited a modest cemetery at the base of Montmartre with one of his friends. This space, commonly known as the Champ de repos, dated from the very end of the eighteenth century when the Department of the Seine created it to replace the popularly reviled cemeteries of Roche and Monceau. Compared to its predecessors, the Champ de repos was a relatively pleasant and picturesque space. And while it was quite small, it featured a wide assortment of tombs, trees, and vegetation that Parisians enjoyed visiting. On this particular day Piétresson de Saint-Aubin and his companion did not seem to mind the Champ de repos's comparatively small size; they were quietly lost in thought, enjoying the somber solitude of the day and the affecting sight of a cemetery blanketed in snow.

Suddenly, the sound of sobbing pulled them out of their reverie. The two men followed the sound to its source and discovered a woman dressed in black, kneeling in the snow before a simple tomb, gripped by "the most profound sorrow."

Piétresson de Saint-Aubin and his friend then engaged in a strange act of communion with this woman—a virtual stranger to them. They were deeply moved by her display of emotion but did not want to "disturb her melancholy" so they kept their distance. Once she left, they approached the tomb and discovered that the object of her sorrow was her sixteen-year-old daughter, Eliza Veroquier, who had died several months earlier. They read Eliza's simple epitaph, which highlighted the mourning mother's heartbreak in its first two lines: "You sleep in peace, my darling, and yet your mother has lost the ability to rest." A fortuitous encounter with some gravediggers then led the pair to discover that this mourning mother had been visiting her daughter's grave with fresh flowers every two days since the girl's burial. Piétresson de Saint-Aubin and his friend were so moved the mother's devotion that they also began to cry and mourn the loss of this sixteen-year-old stranger. Before departing from this "monument to maternal love" the men decided to leave a message for the grieving mother: they used a pencil to inscribe Eliza's tombstone with two poems. When he returned to the tomb a few days later, Piétresson de Saint-Aubin found the mother shedding "tears of pleasure" over their handiwork.[7]

Although no one else admitted to committing such well-intended acts of vandalism, many other early nineteenth-century authors described similarly affecting encounters with unsuspecting mourners in Paris's new cemeteries. For example, in *Promenade sérieuse au cimetière du Père Lachaise,* an author-narrator who went only by the initials "G.G." observed a girl and her younger sister visiting a family tomb with a basket of fresh flowers. He approached the pair of sisters to "spy upon virtue" and silently observed them as they replaced wilted flowers with the new bouquet. Like Piétresson de Saint-Aubin, G.G. felt conflicted by his desire to connect without disrupting. In the end, he restrained his curiosity because he did not want to disturb the "enchanting work" before him.[8] Similarly, when visiting Père Lachaise Cemetery, the prolific travel writer François-Marie Marchant de Beaumont described how his heart filled "with such delicious melancholy" when he observed a widow "flooding

her husband's grave with tears." However, like his fellow cemetery aficionados, Marchant de Beaumont made no attempt to actually approach
the sobbing widow.[9]

Each of these authors reflected, with different degrees of comfort,
the confusing terrain that new cemeteries occupied in early nineteenth-
century Paris. These were municipal public spaces, accessible to anyone during daytime hours, but after the 1804 Imperial Decree they were divided
into ostensibly private plots (concessions). This realized the ideal that so
many reformers had wistfully described in the 1790s, in which anonymous mass graves gave way to individualized sites of commemoration. If
Pierre Dolivier's five-year-old son had died in the early nineteenth, rather
than the late eighteenth century, the despondent father would have known
where to mourn. Yet, as the examples just cited all illustrate, these new
cemeteries were far from private.

These interactions between cemetery aficionados and mourners demonstrate a new kind of sociability that blossomed between the tombstones
of Père Lachaise, characterized by a strange form of intimacy between
strangers who would never meet. By conflating public and private space
in this way, nineteenth-century Parisians took advantage of the cemetery
as a powerful liminal zone in the city. At the most basic level, this was a
fact of geography, since new cemeteries were legally prohibited within
city limits. Once the dead were firmly ensconced in the city's margins they
stopped being a problem for Paris because they no longer posed a threat to
the health and safety of city dwellers. However, as "a sort of antechamber,
between this world and the next," the cemetery also became a powerful
social imaginary.[10] The cemetery did more than blur the distinction between private and public or the boundary between life and death; it also
provided a bridge across the distance between strangers in the postrevolutionary city. In the wake of a Revolutionary period that strained (and
often snapped) traditional bonds of friendship, trust, and loyalty, such
acts of connection reassured cemetery visitors that Paris was capable of
recalibrating its moral compass.[11]

This chapter examines the vibrant new culture of the dead that took
shape in Paris after 1804. In contrast to the small, overcrowded urban
graveyards of the previous century, Paris's new burial spaces offered expansive fields of rest where one could smell blooming trees rather than
decomposing bodies and see hundreds of ordered and maintained private

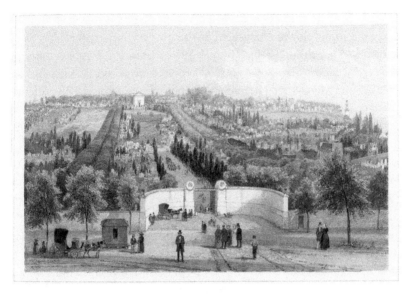

Figure 3.1. J. Jacoltet, "Père Lachaise Cemetery," *Paris et ses environs* (Paris, 1856). The Newberry Library, Chicago (folio G 397.66).

burial plots instead of open mass graves. By the first decade of the nineteenth century, anyone with a free afternoon could travel to the outskirts of Paris and meander through a unique new part of the city whose tombstones and grave markers revealed a diverse population, from famous politicians and artists to the working poor. Régis Bertrand notes that this heterogeneity quickly gave rise to a two-sided commemorative cult of the dead: a public cult for the entombed illustrious elites, and a private cult for the friends and family of the otherwise unknown dead.[12] This chapter challenges that distinction by delving into early nineteenth-century publications that described and analyzed new Parisian cemeteries. As these sources demonstrate, the boundary between public and private was far from clear at the gravesites of ordinary Parisians, like Eliza Veroquier, where private acts of commemoration had a significant impact on a visiting public. Postrevolutionary cemeteries may have lacked the vitrified bones and public death tribunals that ambitious reformers had dreamed up at the end of the eighteenth century, but in their own way they fulfilled the wish that spaces for the dead would become edifying sources of moral and social reconstruction.

The vignettes that opened this chapter all typify a new genre of literature that developed alongside Paris's new cemetery culture. In books with titles that promised picturesque, philosophical, and moral tours of the capital's most macabre spaces, writers like Piétresson de Saint-Aubin, "G.G.," and Marchant de Beaumont combined travel writing with prescriptive moralizing.[13] Most twentieth-century monographs about Père Lachaise and Parisian burial culture make passing reference to these cemetery guidebooks, but they are generally underused by historians, who tend to focus either on the institutional history of cemeteries or their political uses later in the century.[14] However this rich set of sources reveals how contemporary Parisians understood and used their new spaces for the dead to connect with one another in unlikely ways in the postrevolutionary era. Moreover, the authors of these books often expressed their own strong views about what ought (and ought not) to happen inside of a cemetery's walls. The relationship between the cemetery and its visiting public was a conversation that we can uncover and trace through these guidebooks.

Antoine Caillot and the "Language of the Tomb"

The pioneering text for this new genre of cemetery literature was Antoine Caillot's 1808 *Voyage religieux et sentimentale aux quatre cimetières de Paris.* In it, the author—a prolific writer, teacher, and moralist—reconstructed the emotional and physical experience of walking through the city's four operational cemeteries: the Champs de repos at Montmartre (est. 1798), the new Cemetery of the East known as Mont-Louis or Père Lachaise (est. 1804), and two left bank cemeteries that dated from earlier in the eighteenth century, Vaugirard (est. 1793) and Sainte-Catherine (est. 1783). Caillot's *Voyage,* which predated other published cemetery guidebooks by almost a decade, offers a unique view of Parisian cemeteries in a period of transition. Caillot seems to have had one foot in the eighteenth and the other in the nineteenth century. He was at once a critic of cemeteries, an ardent believer in their edifying abilities, and a keen aficionado who could not keep himself away from cemetery gates.

Caillot's book contained both new and familiar themes. Much like the authors of cemetery guidebooks that opened this chapter, Caillot described several of his own vivid encounters with strangers in the cemetery.

For example, toward the end of his lengthy description of Père Lachaise Cemetery, which had only been opened for four years, he came across the elaborately decorated tomb of a twenty-five-year-old woman, Anne-Josephine-Françoise Bontemps. After translating Bontemps's lengthy Latin epitaph, which described a dearly missed daughter, sister, friend, wife, and mother, Caillot recounted his own physical and emotional reaction to the woman's grave. He sat down on the stone bench behind the monument, felt religious awe and sympathy, and attempted to unite his "sighs and regrets" with those of the dead woman's family. He then took this a step further: to "heighten" his grief, he persuaded himself that he had suffered the same "deplorable loss" as Bontemps's family. He recalled happier days and tears began to fall from his eyes. His head dropped down to his chest and he collapsed, overwhelmed by sorrow.[15] Bontemps and her family were complete strangers to Caillot before he happened across her grave, but the simple act of reading and contemplating her tomb compelled him to imagine his way into her life and to vicariously experience her death as though she had been his own much-loved wife or daughter.

Yet, despite this distinctively nineteenth-century scene, Caillot's text also retained a great deal of the previous century's disapproving tone, particularly for the two older burial spaces that he visited and described: the cemeteries of Vaugirard and Sainte-Catherine. These sites occupied a strange place in the emerging nineteenth-century culture of the dead. Although the official plan, as of March 1801, had been to establish three large cemeteries, to the north, south, and east of the city, obtaining large enough tracts of land proved difficult for the Napoleonic State. By 1804 it had only secured the large swath of rural territory to the east of the city, that was commonly referred to as "Mont-Louis" and was known for being the former residence of Louis' XIV's Jesuit confessor Père Lachaise (hence the name). After opening Paris's eastern cemetery, it would take the state another two decades to establish similar spaces to the north and south of the city. Owing to this lag in development, Vaugirard and Sainte-Catherine remained in use as the only cemeteries on Paris's Left Bank until 1824, when they were finally replaced by Montparnasse, a large and modern burial space, in the style of Père Lachaise. The first quarter of the nineteenth century was a period of transition, in which the watershed cemetery of Père Lachaise loomed large over the smaller and shabbier graveyards that lingered from the late eighteenth century.

Like the cemeteries themselves, Caillot's descriptions of Vaugirard and Sainte-Catherine were straight out of the eighteenth century. He invoked familiar tropes of dangerous odors, a dispiriting lack of space, and the "indecent" proximity of the dead to the living. For example, the mass grave at Sainte-Catherine was a "spectacle of desolation" whose "putrid miasmas" endangered the capital. He urged the state to close both of these unfortunate cemeteries as soon as possible.[16] These kinds of complaints about outdated cemeteries would have easily made up the bulk of any eighteenth-century pamphlet about French burial practices, but times had changed and they only appeared in the last twenty pages of Caillot's 355-page book. Instead, most of his narrative was dedicated to re-creating the visual, emotional, and mental experience of visiting Paris's two newest cemeteries: the Champ de repos at Montmartre and the expansive new Cemetery of the East, Père Lachaise.

At the time of Caillot's writing, Père Lachaise Cemetery was only four years old and not yet an overbearing presence that dominated every depiction and discussion of French cemeteries. The "Maison du Père La Chaise à Mont-Louis" did not even make an appearance until almost halfway through Caillot's *Voyage*. Instead, the first and most detailed section of the book was devoted to the (slightly) more established cemetery located at the base of Montmartre. Although the Champ de repos would be expanded to almost 30 acres in 1825, in 1808 this cemetery was barely a tenth of that size, 3.14 acres. By comparison, Père Lachaise comprised 43.4 acres in 1804 and was expanded to 56.8 in 1824. Thus, when Caillot visited the Champ de repos it occupied a middle ground in Paris's cemetery revolution: it was not as reviled as Vaugirard and Sainte-Catherine, but neither was it up to the new standard of Père Lachaise. Perhaps because of this association with the city's older cemetery culture, Caillot's description of the Champ de repos employed the eighteenth-century technique of using a cemetery to critique the capital's social and moral health.

Caillot began his narrative on a dark and stormy day, when his somber and melancholy thoughts drew him to the front gate of the Champ de repos. From the very beginning of his narrative, however, Caillot kept a wary eye on the community that surrounded the cemetery. In particular, he expressed concern about the nearby fashionable neighborhood of the Chaussée-d'Antin, where he imagined the *nouveaux riches* counting their money, the poor exploiting themselves, and passionate young men spending too much time cavorting in salons and cafés. "Young man," the author cautioned, "you would do well to leave the salons of the Chaussée-d'Antin from time to time and take a walk through the Champ de repos."[17] Specifically, he suggested that his imagined reader ought to spend a few moments sitting in the cemetery and contemplating the graves of so many of his peers. In fact, the numerous graves of young people in Montmartre perplexed and concerned Caillot. Naturally, he found the premature deaths of so many Parisians deeply saddening and proclaimed that the whole of society owed these young people "torrents" of tears. But he also expressed great anxiety over the meaning of so many early deaths, which he interpreted as evidence of a generation corrupted by self-interest and hedonistic pursuits. For example, after reading the headstone of a twenty-three-year-old woman, he warned "cheeky" and "lighthearted" women that living their lives only for pleasure would lead them to an early grave. He was similarly concerned about the number of young men buried in Montmartre, whose deaths he attributed to their propensity to consume rich foods, drink dangerous liquors, and attend too many night-time spectacles and parties.[18]

These concerns about a dangerously frivolous young Paris recalls anxieties of the 1790s, when cemetery reformers had collectively wrung their hands about the degraded moral character of Parisians after the Terror. Caillot, too, remained vexed about the long-term effects of "a bloody revolution that left so much excess in its wake; that animated hatreds, excited vengeance, and broke or loosened all the reins of society."[19] This passing reference to the social chaos that the Revolution allegedly left behind also appears in Caillot's two-volume history of Parisian moeurs, published two decades later toward the end of the Restoration. In it, he reiterated his assessment of early nineteenth-century Paris as a hedonistic, immoral, and irreligious city, replete with orgies and nude swimmers in the Seine![20] Although concerns about social and moral collapse were on the wane after the institution of the Napoleonic Empire and the stability that it represented, France in the first decade of the nineteenth century retained the aura of decadence and instability that it had gained during the 1790s.[21] Indeed, in 1808, the same year that Caillot published his cemetery book, the Académie de Dijon asked their correspondents: "Does the French nation deserve the reputation for fickleness that it has with foreigners?"[22]

For Caillot, this unhealthy pursuit of pleasure was closely linked to the dangerous scourge of "materialism" (meaning, atheism) that lingered from the Revolutionary period. Although he was ultimately soothed by the number of religious symbols and messages present in Paris's municipal cemeteries, Caillot—a devout Catholic—also used his description of the Champ de repos to air his concerns about a population without religion. At the end of his third day touring Montmartre, Caillot decided to take advantage of good weather and (secretly) spend the night alone in the cemetery. After settling in for the night and overcoming a brief fit of terror, Caillot described feeling overwhelmed by a profound sense of awe and appreciation for the truth, wisdom, and eloquence that was engraved on the stones that surrounded him. He exalted this "language of the tomb" as the surrogate voice of the silent dead.[23] Halfway through his macabre slumber party the dead spoke to Caillot even more directly, when a desolate ghost dressed only in a burial shroud, appeared before him and began to speak. The ghost explained how, as an eighteenth-century adolescent he had regrettably fallen prey to the "pointless sophisms" of "so-called philosophes." As punishment, he was forced to endure complete isolation after death, with nothing but his tortured thoughts to keep him company, which he described as "the greatest torture that an immortal spirit can endure."[24]

This imaginary encounter with the atheist ghost reveals two important themes in Caillot's narrative. First, as the title of his book indicates, Caillot's *Voyage* was both sentimental and religious. His anxiety about the immoral and wayward youth of Napoleonic Paris was accented by his concern about the place of Christianity in the Empire. Although by 1808, Napoleon had ostensibly reconciled with the Catholic Church, the city's cemeteries remained an ambiguously sacred space: they were administered jointly by the church and state, but they remained civic spaces where people of all faiths and philosophies (including atheism) were officially welcomed. However, this spectral dialogue also demonstrates the persistence of eighteenth-century optimism about the curative properties of well-organized cemeteries. Even someone as desperate and desolate as the atheist ghost experienced redemption when, at the end of his conversation with Caillot, he turned his face toward the sky and disappeared.

Similarly, although Caillot was deeply unsettled by the graves of so many young people, he also saw them as a valuable prophylactic against the degradation of Parisian moeurs. For example, after coming across the tomb of a twenty-eight-year-old man, Caillot directly addressed all the young men who may have been similarly led astray in recent years: "You may turn a deaf ear to the sermons of moralists, but listen closely to the language of the tomb." Caillot similarly invoked the "language of the mausoleum" when describing the tomb of a sixteen-year-old girl. "It is up to me," he explained, "to instruct and frighten these people, because I speak to them in the language of the casket, and I reveal to them the open tombs that will be the end result of all their parties, pleasures, fashions, luxury, recklessness, and excess."[25] Clearly, for Caillot cemeteries did more than bear witness to the problems of the generation who came of age after 1789; they also provided a useful and updated memento mori to shock their visitors into more socially constructive behavior. In this way, his observations retained the reform-minded spirit of the 1790s, whereby the cemetery fulfilled a valuable social function: it brought people together, urged them to contemplate their own mortality, and ideally shaped them into more productive and moral members of society. Significantly, however, it was not just the sight of the tombs and proximity to death that accomplished this transformation, it was also the specific act of reading and contemplating epitaphs, whether as warnings or as models of good behavior. Indeed, in the book's forward Caillot explained his motivation for writing as a desire to share with his audience the important virtues inscribed on stone, including "maternal tenderness, conjugal fidelity, friendship, probity, selflessness, temperance, justice, [and] benevolence."[26]

In the service of this project, Caillot offered abundant examples of virtuous citizens, whose domestic and professional virtues were communicated using the eloquent "language of the tomb." It was this anthologizing aspect of his work that attracted the most attention from his contemporaries. A negative review in the *Mercure de France* criticized Caillot's tone and overt moralizing but admitted that the book was "an enterprise not without utility." The critic concluded: "This book is interesting; it was impossible for it not to be, but it bears repeating that the only thing worth recommending in this book are the epitaphs that it contains."[27] Caillot certainly agreed about the edifying nature of epitaphs; as he wrote halfway through his book: "I think and learn more in front of a tomb and reading an epitaph, than from the most beautiful books in the Imperial Library."[28]

"The Superb City of the Dead" at Père Lachaise

The level of detail in Caillot's description as well as his idiosyncratic commentary set the standard for books about Paris's burgeoning cemetery culture. Although his was the only book about Parisian cemeteries that was available during the Napoleonic Empire, several new publications joined it after the Bourbon Restoration. Pierre-François Piétresson de Saint-Aubin's 1816 *Promenade* through Parisian burial spaces (expanded and republished in 1825) and C. P. Arnaud's two-volume 1817 *Recueil de tombeaux* both detailed the capital's multiple burial spaces, in the model of Caillot's *Voyage*. However, after 1816 more authors began to focus on the singularity of Père Lachaise. For example, the comprehensive compilation by the Rogers (father and son) documented every one of the 2,092 tombs and epitaphs that stood in Père Lachaise Cemetery as of 1816. The prolific conservative travel writer François-Marie Marchant de Beaumont began publishing about Père Lachaise in 1820 and republished variations on the same book under slightly different names at least six times between 1820 and 1828. Other books, like L. E. Chennechot's *Promenades philosophiques et sentimentales au cimetière du Père La Chaise* (1823), Jean-Pons-Guillaume Viennet's *Promenade philosophique au cimetière du Père La Chaise* (1824), or G.G.'s aforementioned *Promenade sérieuse* (1826) were for sale only briefly and remain scant in libraries and archives throughout the world. Whether obscure or best-selling, these guidebooks are all useful sources that provide a thorough record of tombs and epitaphs that have long since disappeared. Just as valuably, they offer a compendium of contemporary reactions to these sites.

While epitaphs and tombs had been in use for centuries in Paris, their quantity and quality changed dramatically in the early nineteenth century.[29] A new genre of tombstone inscription, the long-format biographical epitaph, exemplified this change. These lengthy inscriptions contained significantly more than just names and dates: they often covered a range of personal and professional information about the deceased, more reminiscent of obituaries than epitaphs. For example, Regnault de Saint-Jean d'Angély commissioned a mausoleum topped with both a cenotaph and a cinerary urn to commemorate his death. The monument was covered in clearly engraved bronze inscriptions, which provided a chronological list of all of Regnault's important accomplishment and setbacks. From this list, one learned not only about his birth and death, but also about his election to the constituent assembly (in 1789), his proscription (in 1794), his various promotions in the Napoleonic State (1799–1815), and the exile (1815) that may have eventually led to his death (1819). As one author who drew and described the tomb noted, "What more could we add to the story of M. le compte Regnault de Saint-Jean d'Angély's life? Everything is written out on his tomb."[30]

For the overwhelming majority of the population who did not live such eventful lives, tombstones were an opportunity to demonstrate the virtues of their domestic and private lives. This reinforces the argument that many historians have made about how ostensibly private relationships between friends, families, and lovers became important sources of social cohesion in the early nineteenth century.[31] Epitaphs for both men and women constantly commended the deceased for being excellent spouses, parents, and friends. For example, Antoine Albaret's tomb (1750–1813) proclaimed that anyone who took his life as a model ("good since childhood, he never wavered, he was a good husband and father") would find happiness.[32] It was very common to describe a woman as "an example of virtue . . . the best of wives and the most sincere of friends"[33] or a man as "the best of husbands, the tenderest of fathers, and the most sincere of friends."[34] In 1825 Jacques-Antoine Dulaure interpreted these epitaphs as evidence that "public morality" had made great progress since the Old Regime. "Previously," he explained "we would have thought it better to commend the dead not for his virtues, but for his titles, his dignities, and the signs of his power, but such feudal pride is in short supply at Père Lachaise."[35] Others were less sanguine, such as François-Marie Marchant de Beaumont, who noted that if one judged by the contents of Parisian epitaphs, the capital was populated only by good parents, excellent spouses, and perfect friends. Everyone seemed to have become flawless as soon as they entered the tomb, he wryly noted.[36] Similarly, M. Roger and his son made the epigram to their 1816 book: "How many lies on all of these stones!"[37]

Up until the early nineteenth century, such "lies" would generally have only been possible for the very wealthy or well known. However, landmark legislation in the early years of the Empire made this new epitaph culture accessible to a wider range of Parisians. When the Napoleonic State issued its decree on burial practices just days after the first burial took place in Père Lachaise in June 1804, one of the most revolutionary features of this decree was its commitment to providing a unique grave for each deceased individual. It guaranteed each deceased body their own space in the ground, separated from their neighbor by at least thirty centimeters. The style and permanence of each gravesite would vary depending on how much money the family and ancestors of the deceased were willing to pay. The small size of Paris's pre-1804 cemeteries (Montmartre, Vaugirard, and Sainte-Catherine) did not allow for total compliance with the new regulations, but since Père Lachaise was the first Parisian cemetery of the new era, the prefecture of the Seine organized the territory at Mont-Louis in accordance with the new regulations. The entire cemetery was surrounded by a large stone wall, to prevent animals and undesirable people from misusing the space. Within the walled-in area, special sections were reserved for religious minorities and the rest of the cemetery was divided up according to wealth. The terrain along the southwestern wall of the cemetery was designated as "public," where the poor could be buried free of charge in a communal grave. The remainder of the vast expanse was intended for permanent and semipermanent gravesites for individuals and families who were able and willing to pay the set fees.[38] Individuals who buried family members in the "public" cemetery were guaranteed the same spot for at least six years and were permitted to erect temporary markers or plant gardens as they saw fit. Additional laws and regulations continually upheld the burial rights of "indigents" and the hierarchical organization of burial practices.[39]

At the opposite extreme from the communal grave were "perpetual concessions" that one could purchase for the steep price of one hundred francs per square meter (with a two square meter minimum). A perpetual concession guaranteed a permanent place in the cemetery that could be embellished according to the owner's means and desires. The concept that a portion of the public cemetery could be privately purchased was unprecedented and revolutionary; within a generation it gave rise to Père Lachaise's unique array of elaborate and picturesque tombs that commemorated wealthy or notable individuals and families. For certain famous figures, such as the poet Jacques Delille, groups would raise funds for a perpetual concession through a subscription service, which lent an air of community to even the most "private" of property at Père Lachaise. From 1804 until 1824, Père Lachaise was the only cemetery in France that accommodated permanent concessions, but this practice quickly spread to later cemeteries, like Montparnasse Cemetery (est. 1824) and the renovated and expanded cemetery at Montmartre (est. 1825).

There was also a third burial option. For individuals who wanted something more private than the mass grave, but who could not afford the exclusive private plots, Père Lachaise offered "temporary concessions" that could be rented rather than purchased. By 1825 these temporary concessions were limited to five years each, after which point families had the option to either upgrade to permanent concessions or have the deceased moved to the communal grave. Although this intermediary option was relatively accessible and attractive to much of the Parisian population, by the 1820s, concessions, whether permanent or temporary, comprised only a fraction of burials. According to the *Recherches statistiques sur la ville de Paris,* between 1821 and 1823, 13.2 percent of annual burials were temporary concessions and a slim 4.4 percent were permanent, leaving a large majority of 82.2 percent buried free of charge in the communal grave.[40] The number of concessions would increase throughout the nineteenth century, but as late as 1875, 63 percent burials still took place in the common grave, with 10 percent in permanent concessions, and 27 percent in temporary concessions.[41]

Despite this stratified structure, contemporary authors and critics regularly interpreted Père Lachaise Cemetery as a profoundly unifying and cohesive space. It brought strangers into contact in one another, reunited loved ones beyond the tomb, and resolved the rift between the city and its dead that had for years caused so much distress. Throughout the late eighteenth century poorly maintained cemeteries had been widely interpreted as evidence of Parisian degradation. By contrast, the hyperbolic attention that Parisians paid to the dead in spaces like Père Lachaise was a way to rebuild sociability and demonstrate how far Parisian moeurs had come since the 1790s. As Marchant de Beaumont explained it in 1821, during the Old Regime, "an insurmountable barrier" had separated the living and the dead. The Revolution successfully destroyed that barrier, but it also shattered "all the bonds of nature" and reduced cemeteries to "fields of carnage." Père Lachaise resolved both of these problems, since it had "nothing of the somber character of Paris's old cemeteries" and acted as "a superb city of the dead, placed between the limits of both worlds" where the power of memories united the past with the present and brought life and death together.[42] Significantly, this theme of reunion did not only refer to the traditional expectation of a heavenly reunion of souls after death, but to the literal intermingling of human remains in the newly sacred space of the municipal cemetery.

Cemetery Sociability

There were many tombs in Père Lachaise that provided evidence of post-mortem reunions. Arguably the most famous attraction at Père Lachaise after 1817 was the recently constructed chapel that contained the reunited bones of the famously ill-fated medieval lovers, Abélard and Héloïse. However, this same spirit of Romantic reunion proliferated among the ordinary dead, such as the conjoined graves of Marie-Anne Maroy and her spouse J. B. Réveillon. Maroy's epitaph ended with Réveillon's exhortation about the injustice of not being able to die as he had lived—alongside his wife. When Réveillon died two years later, his epitaph explained how "he truly ceased living the day that [Marie-Anne] was taken from him. All of his affections, all of his thoughts were with her" and his "only desire" since her death had been to join her in the tomb as soon as possible.[43] A similar fate befell Mme Atrof, who died in 1807 after losing her two young daughters to illness in 1805 and 1806. Atrof's grief was apparently so extreme, that nothing, not even her husband's love could revive her. She languished in a depressed state for a year and a half before she finally died happy that she would be buried in the same tomb as her daughters.[44] We know all of this detail about Atrof, Maroy, and Réveillon because of their epitaphs, which detailed their tragic biographies.

Other aspirational epitaphs referenced these types of reunions in the tomb as a wish for the future. For example, Sophie Hédé's epitaph read:

Here rests forever Dame Marie-Thérèse-Sophie Hédé. Widow to Louis-Eustache Poitier Delille and wife to Mr. Charles-Marie-Jacques-Joseph-Gaspart Tutot, deceased the 30th of July 1813. Time will reunite us, dear Sophie, and your poor Charles will finally stop being miserable. You were a good mother, you will live forever in the heart of your children.[45]

Similarly, after seventeen-year-old Alexandre-Hector Lemaire died, his parents engraved a large marble vase with gold lettering and promised to join him in the tomb before too long:

Those who should have preceded you in the tomb will soon rest near to you, one on your right, the other on your left; this father, who . . . cannot escape his pain and this most miserable of all mothers, inconsolable because there is nothing in the world that can comfort her now that you are gone.[46]

By this point, it should be clear that early nineteenth-century epitaphs were only in part about the individuals that they ostensibly commemorated. Supportive individuals from the deceased's circle of friends and family, like Mme Atrof's helpless husband or Lemaire's desolate parents, often made subtle (and not-so-subtle) appearances in epitaphs. Even when these individuals were not overtly wishing for their own deaths, surviving friends and family members regularly appeared as active participants. For example, André-Louis-Etienne Bray's epitaph explained that "his family and friends, who will never stop missing him, erected this little monument to his memory."[47] Similarly, Louis-Clarion-Gustave Bethfort's tomb was inscribed as a "monument to the pain of an inconsolable mother and father" who promised to "cry forever" for their lost son.[48] These types of epitaphs abounded in Père Lachaise; one can hardly turn a page in the Rogers' 1816 catalog of the cemetery without coming across multiple references to suffering survivors. Just a cursory sample includes the following:

Here rests Charles-Edouard Delaroche, born the 18th of November, 1741, deceased the 20th of December 1813. The best of husbands, the most tender of fathers; his heart was the sanctuary for every virtue. His widow, who shared 32 years of happiness with him, and his inconsolable children will visit and cry over his tomb for the rest of their lives.[49]

Here lies Louis-Jean-Baptiste Nores, died on 25 May, 1815, aged 60 years and 4 months. The tenderness of his widow [and] the regret and piety of his children have erected for him this monument of their sharp and perpetual pain.[50]

The body of Marie-Anne Chardon, widow of Alexandre Duhamel, former wine seller, deceased at the age of 75 years and 9 months, at 39 rue St. Bernard, on the 8th of April, 1813. The loss of this respectable mother was a calamity for her children, who cried as much after her death as they cherished her during her life.[51]

To the most cherished of wives and the best of mothers.
Here lies Marie-Cecile Bigot, wife of Jean-Julie Guenin, former drink seller,
    deceased on May 6, 1814 aged 42 years.
She is no more! In their bitter pain,
A husband and nine children will cry for her every day:
She was their hope, their joy, and their love.
Oh! There is no more happiness on earth for them.
Pray to God for her.[52]

One of the most notable early tombs from Père Lachaise was that of Antoine de Guillaume Lagrange (figure 3.2). Lagrange was a cavalry solider (*dragon*) in the Napoleonic army who died on the battlefield in Poland in 1807 when he was twenty-five years old. A year later, his mother had a cenotaph erected in his honor that featured his face in relief. Because it was the first tomb that featured a sculptural effigy, it attracted attention, and throughout the Restoration Lagrange's tomb became a gathering place for veterans of the Napoleonic wars. It was such a prominent attraction in Père Lachaise that the main path on which it stands is still known as the *chemin du dragon* (path of the dragoon). The content of Lagrange's epitaph is as noteworthy as its appearance: it stands as an excellent example of an early nineteenth-century attestation of grief. Every surface of the monument was covered with narrative details about his life and death, but it also contains an unexpected level of detail about his surviving mother. At the top of its inscription, the cenotaph was introduced as an "homage of a tender mother to the memory of the best and most unfortunate of sons." Reading on, one learns that Lagrange was an only child, that he died a hero, and that he was missed by "his superiors, his friends, his colleagues, and generally everyone who knew him." The intimate details of his death were also etched in stone:

> After having proven his worth at Austerlitz, Jéna, and Erfurth, etc. he found death in the terrifying deserts of Poland in combat on the 4th of February, 1807; it happened in a dangerous passage at the entry point to a village. When it was asked who would lead the charge he immediately volunteered . . . he threw himself forward and a bullet instantly pierced his heart! His final words on the battlefield were: "My mother! My poor mother!"

The epitaph then shifts from the descriptive to the personal, and from the third to the first person: "Oh my dear and beloved son! My best friend! The most precious thing in the world to me! . . . Only death itself will bring my suffering to an end."[53]

Among contemporaries, Mme Lagrange's engraved suffering was generally well received. In his 1817 *Recueil de tombeaux*, C. P. Arnaud devoted three pages of his book to a description of the cenotaph, moved by the inscriptions he called "proof of the most exalted pain."[54] In Arnaud's opinion, the cenotaph was the product of Mme Lagrange's "pious and very legitimate melancholy." He further remarked that it was one of the most effective monuments in the cemetery because it inspired "consoling emotions" and reminded passersby of the "precious virtues" that were in regrettably short supply among the general population, virtues such as "maternal love, filial piety, conjugal fidelity, appreciation [reconnaissance] etc. etc."[55] Similarly, after describing and transcribing the cenotaph, François-Marie Marchant de Beaumont called on every mother who lost a son to visit the Lagrange monument, to mix their tears with those of Mme Lagrange, and to follow her model and erect memorials to their lost sons.[56]

As Arnaud and Marchant de Beaumont's reactions illustrate, this grief etched in stone was far from a one-sided performance. The reunions taking place in Père Lachaise were emphatically not limited to families and friends. Although tombs and epitaphs occupied "private" space (whether purchased or rented), they cannot be read as simple intimate expressions of sorrow: they were written for an audience. Some epitaphs

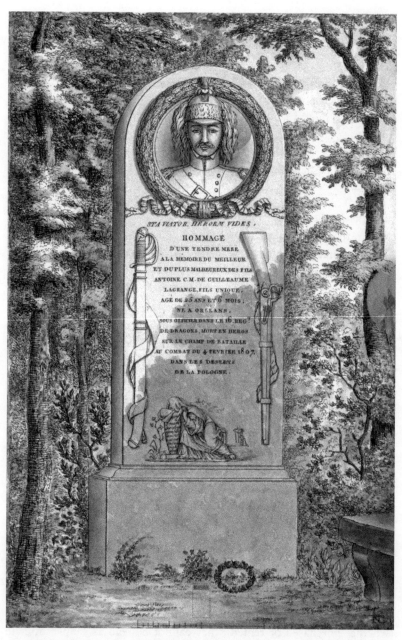

Figure 3.2. C. P. Arnaud, "Tomb of Antoine Lagrange," *Recueil des quatre cimetières de Paris* (Paris, 1817).

were more direct about the public nature of their work. For example, Antoine-André Bavrio, a poet and artist used his tombstone to announce that his estate would award three thousand francs to the first person who discovered a cure for the mercury sickness that afflicted so many gilders.[57] Many other epitaphs made similarly specific demands of their audience by requesting tears, sympathy, prayers, or flowers. If epitaphs spoke the "language of the tomb," the conversations they sought were frequently with strangers.

The nineteenth-century obsession with the tomb has conventionally been interpreted as evidence of the growing strength of the bourgeois family and its emphasis on sentimental love.[58] In this reading, most famously articulated by Philippe Ariès, the gravesite became an extension of the home and an opportunity to prolong relationships after death. However, a closer examination of early nineteenth-century tombs and their inscriptions reveals a persistent attempt to establish bonds beyond immediate circles of friends and family. In new spaces that blurred the distinction between private and public, a kind of cemetery sociability began to flourish. Epitaphs conveyed ostensibly private emotions to an anonymous public, who visited cemeteries to connect with their fellow Parisians, both living and dead. The authors of cemetery guidebooks then translated and annotated this experience into words and images for their reading audience, who could replicate these sentiments at home.

Borrowed Space

New burial spaces like Père Lachaise were well received in the early nineteenth century in part because they stood in such stark contrast to what came before them. Rather than offering visitors the unpleasant sight (and smell) of decomposing bodies intermingling in an open mass grave, Père Lachaise promised flowering trees, green bushes, and beautiful stone grave markers. Pierre-François Piétresson de Saint-Aubin described how the rest of Europe was astonished by the cemetery's "diversity of monuments . . . the variety of their distribution, the little gardens that surround them, and the trees that hang over them and provide shade."[59] Indeed, the kind of cemetery guidebook that Piétresson de Saint-Aubin published—a descriptive account of the author's edifying promenades through Parisian burial spaces—would not have been possible a decade earlier, when the only publications about French cemeteries were dedicated to their wholesale renovation. As we have seen, these Empire- and Restoration-era cemetery guidebooks were overwhelmingly concerned with the details of individual graves and epitaphs. However, such emphasis on Père Lachaise's innovative structure and appearance obscured the fact that by 1821, more than 80 percent of burials at Père Lachaise took place in the communal grave. Most authors made little or no mention of this, and those that did made a point of explaining how dramatically the communal grave at Père Lachaise differed from those of the eighteenth century.

In his 1817 publication *Recueil des tombeaux des quatre cimetières de Paris*, C. P. Arnaud addressed the communal graves in Père Lachaise in glowing terms. He described a series of long trenches, approximately six feet deep, that ran parallel to the rest of the cemetery. Gravediggers, he emphasized, placed the dead side by side in their coffins rather than on top of one another, as had previously been the custom. As each trench filled, another was dug, which was possible because of Père Lachaise's forty-acre expanse. Owing to the lack of crowding, bodies decomposed fairly quickly, which meant each trench could be renewed after five or six years. Arnaud also described an unexpected, but appreciated, consequence of this successful management: the ground surrounding the communal graves was extremely fertile and featured the thickest and most "startlingly green" grass in all of the cemetery. In contrast to this lush productivity, Arnaud described the Vaugirard Cemetery (which dated back to 1793) as a fetid hole exhaling dangerous and "putrid miasmas" into the atmosphere. He found Montmartre's cemetery slightly less problematic, since it used the same trench-style graves as Père Lachaise, but because of its much smaller terrain (before 1825), gravediggers were unfortunately forced to stack the dead on top of one another in a twelve-to-fifteen foot trench.[60]

Beyond its novel and hygienic mode of burial, Père Lachaise's mass graves also appealed to some authors because they made it possible for the poor and the wealthy to honor their dead in the same way: by erecting monuments on the very spot that their loved one lay buried. The Rogers' 1816 compendium of the tombs at Père Lachaise provided an overview of these markers in the communal grave, which were for the most part simple wooden crosses adorned with the deceased's name along with their date of birth and death, although on occasion they featured short inscriptions such as, "Everyone who knew him has cried for him. He leaves behind an inconsolable brother" or "Rest in peace sweet child, you'll never know your mother and father's pain."[61] Some family members who used the communal grave also took advantage of their temporary cemetery real estate to plant small gardens surrounded by little fences to demarcate a loved one's final resting place. These temporary markers kept with the basic principles of the 1804 Imperial Decree, which guaranteed each individual the right to be buried in her or his own grave. It also maintained the unique appeal and usefulness of Père Lachaise as a cemetery that celebrated the inspiring achievements of individuals. In comparison, the communal grave at Vaugirard seemed like a regrettable waste of "good fathers, virtuous mothers, [and] loyal spouses" who could have served as examples "to all social classes," but were destined to be forgotten in the anonymous pit, as one author lamented.[62] By extending the "tomb cult" to the communal grave, Père Lachaise rectified this presumed injustice. Finally, by providing the poor and the wealthy with a similar experience, Père Lachaise offered tangible evidence that supported the conventional wisdom that everyone was equal in death. Arnaud delighted in this fact, announcing in the preface to his book that new cemeteries provided at long last a solution to the "chimera of equality" because "in the night of the tomb: equality is perfect."[63]

Arnaud's romantic notion of the cemetery's egalitarianism found a corollary in other cemetery guidebooks whose authors glorified and admired the poor for their virtuous behavior in Père Lachaise. This valorization appeared most strongly in François-Marie Marchant de Beaumont's descriptions of Père Lachaise from the early 1820s. In at least two different publications, he described witnessing the burial of a twelve-year-old girl in the "popular cemetery." The episode, which varied slightly in different editions of his books, featured the girl's father and her younger brother and sister. Marchant de Beaumont focused his reader's attention on how the two children held hands and wept uncontrollably throughout the procession, while their hard-working father's face revealed "the most profound pain." The little sister eventually collapsed under the emotional weight of the day and her father had to carry her "almost lifeless" body out of the cemetery. Marchant de Beaumont immediately interrogated his own emotional response after recounting this "touching scene." He explained that what he saw had penetrated his heart; the young family's desolation completely overwhelmed his senses.[64] In the slightly more elaborate version of this story, Marchant de Beaumont concluded his emotional analysis by imagining the occupants of the communal grave speaking to him with one voice: "We lived poor, without consideration or credit in the world that you now inhabit" they announced from beyond the tomb. They then provided him with some otherworldly advice and reminded him that a life spent in pursuit of "fickle and fleeting pleasures" would lead to "certain and ceaseless unhappiness" because in the afterlife "only virtue obtains the immortal crown."[65]

It is difficult not to read these sentimental acclamations of the mass grave at Père Lachaise as disingenuous. For someone like Marchant de Beaumont, the deceased poor were most useful as a ghostly memento mori for his wealthy audience, reminding them to live virtuous and unselfish lives. This becomes even more evident when we examine the broader context in which he discussed the communal grave. In both of the books cited above, he introduced the city's poor to act as a foil to the post-revolutionary nouveaux riches. Indeed, immediately prior to describing the "touching" family funeral scene, Marchant de Beaumont recounted a horrific episode that read like a scene straight out of a Balzac novel. In it, a wealthy property owner negotiated the cost of a funeral monument for his relative, for whom he had purchased a temporary concession. The savvy shopper initially requested a beautiful monument worthy of his virtuous relative but balked at each of the marble setter's suggestions on the grounds that they were too "pompous" for his simple, frugal, and philosophical relative. He finally settled on the smallest stone with the shortest possible inscription, all at a below-market price. At the conclusion of this negotiation, the wealthy man rubbed his hands together with greedy glee, excited that he would soon be able to tell everyone that he'd buried his relative in Père Lachaise. After observing this scene, Marchant de Beaumont walked off in an indignant huff and contemplated the deplorable moral state of his beloved Paris,

> a city where everyone is so concerned with themselves, and so little with others; where everyone works for their own fortune, sacrifices everything for

their own pleasure; where modest virtue hides and vanity glows brightly; where daily one witnesses death and funerals, but barely thinks about one's own impending death.

Immediately after this lament, Marchant de Beaumont looked up to find himself at the edge of the "popular cemetery," where the twelve-year-old girl's funeral was in process. "Let us see," he remarked, "if the poor are equally devoid of affective sentiment." In his interpretation, as we have already seen, they were not.[66]

With his moral condemnation of the greedy rich, Marchant de Beaumont updated the postrevolutionary trope of using cemetery behavior as evidence of social decay. The most dangerous villains in his books were not godless materialists, disrespectful porters, or hedonistic party people, but the self-interested rich who, like the scheming bourgeois described above, valued appearances over substance. These types of characters, who reappear several times in Marchant de Beaumont's travel narratives, purchased temporary concessions when they had the means to afford perpetual ones and spent lavishly on ostentatious funeral performances rather than investing in permanent resting places for their family and friends. Marchant de Beaumont implored his wealthy readers not to needlessly condemn their loved ones to "borrowed graves":

> Do not disregard their remains, they should be dear to your heart; do not permit them this most cruel insult, do not allow them to entirely disappear from the earth. Rescue them from this disgrace and free yourself from shame. If you are a father, make it possible for your children to cry over their ancestors' tomb and at their mother's coffin; do not deprive them of this sad relief. Set a pious example and they will repay you by providing a similarly permanent home for your remains. . . . The government has fulfilled its duties, now it is up to you to honor the debt of blood, of friendship, and of recognition.[67]

This "advice" not to scrimp on funereal real estate reveals much about the important place that the cemetery had come to occupy in Paris by the 1820s. Most obviously, it provided a permanent and personalized resting place that acted as a vital link across time. However, this passage also clearly reiterates the belief that dominated so many cemetery reform proposals of the 1790s: that being forgotten after death was the worst punishment one could suffer, and that the population (and the state) had a moral obligation to ensure that this would not happen. Much earlier in the century, Antoine Caillot also invoked this sentiment when he wondered why the epitaphs he encountered in Parisian cemeteries seemed overwhelmingly positive. "Where are all the wives who tortured their husbands and made them miserable?" he asked; "Ah! Without a doubt they have been condemned to the communal grave . . ."[68] In this formulation, temporary burial places, whether in the communal grave or in five-year concessions were roughly equivalent to Thomas Doderet's 1800 "black cemetery" or General Pommereul's "field of oblivion." However, to nineteenth-century commentators like Marchant de Beaumont, a five-year grave undermined the cohesive social function of cemeteries: it not only deprived the deceased of their eternal home, it also prevented them from connecting with future generations. "Borrowed," graves also belied the optimistic narrative that postrevolutionary Parisians had overcome the dangerous indifference toward the dead that had raised so many hackles at the end of the eighteenth century.

How can we square this hostility toward temporary burial spaces with the praise that men like Marchant de Beaumont showered on the grieving poor? The answer most likely lies in his presumably wealthy readership. Whenever he addressed his audience directly, Marchant de Beaumont assumed they were Parisians of means. In his book the poor were reduced to sympathetic families, doing all that they could to honor the dead. This filial devotion modeled the sentiment—if not the practice—that he sought to encourage among his readers. Indeed, the very last paragraph in his 426-page book urged his readers to visit "the last residence of the poor," which he promised would be even more moving and satisfying to sensitive hearts than the most superb private monuments in the cemetery.[69] With this kind of statement that privileged moral rather than material wealth, Marchant de Beaumont was reasserting the "perfect equality" that Arnaud had praised several years earlier. If it seemed to these observers that the city was becoming increasingly stratified by wealth, the cemetery could offer some perspective and recalibrate these differences. The Rogers noted as much in their two-volume catalog of every tomb in Père Lachaise, as of 1816. They explained how effectively the new cemetery hosted the remains of all of Parisians: children, warriors, savants, and humble artisans all lay together: elaborate monuments stood in close proximity to humble graves, but all deserved and received the same pious respect from the sensitive souls who visited the cemetery.[70]

The Limits of Père Lachaise

In 1814 Alexandre-Théodore Brogniart, the son of Père Lachaise's architect, described his father's design as a space that had to navigate a series of contrasts: "nobility without magnificence, and simplicity without negligence." It also needed to inspire "religious sentiment without terror," "respect without sadness" and convey "a sort of melancholy charm, resulting from the nature and arrangement of its monuments."[71] This quote illustrates one of the most useful accomplishments of Paris's new cemetery: its ability to unite the city's disparate population together under the aegis of mourning. After a decade of confusion and chaos, this "superb city of the dead" provided each individual with a place to mourn their dead and offered the public a front-row seat to this satisfying spectacle. And in contrast to the complex and tumultuous city that it served, the "Paris" on display in Père Lachaise was relatively easy to understand. By visiting (or reading about) the cemetery, one could empathize equally with a wealthy mother who had erected an elaborate tomb to her dead son, or impoverished children who visited their father in the communal grave. But this lofty notion of emotional equivalence breaks down under scrutiny. In contrast to the wealthy mother, who knew for certain that her son lay in his private concession (whether temporary or perpetual), the poor family may actually have been mourning in the wrong place.

After thirty years of operation, the state examined Paris's communal burial practices and concluded that, contrary to the initial plan of 1804, the goal of providing each Parisian with their own recognizable grave was not always being met. The difficulty began at the point of burial, where coffins in the communal trenches were placed slightly closer together than expected. This became particularly problematic when mourners marked out their individual portion of the mass grave using fences or gardens; these demarcations were usually several inches wider than the space actually allotted to each coffin. When compounded several times over in the same trench, this quickly led to misaligned gravestones. An 1837 report about the history of this problem offered the example of a picturesque little garden in the communal cemetery that a devoted mother had been carefully maintaining over her daughter's presumed grave. An exhumation revealed that the body beneath the garden was that of a young man, while the girl's remains were actually located three coffins further down the trench.[72] The vaunted "equality in death" that guidebook authors observed in Père Lachaise was a consoling narrative, but it was ultimately an illusion. If Parisians wanted to access a city space where the dead were truly equal, they needed to write a letter to the General Inspector of Mines and Quarries and request a ticket of entry into the Paris Catacombs.

4

The Empire of the Dead

As Père Lachaise was developing into one of Paris's most picturesque and macabre destinations, increasing numbers of Parisians and foreigners met on the southern edge of the city to tour another new space for the dead. There, at the (coincidentally, but aptly named) Barrière d'enfer they met, armed with admission tickets, candles, and curiosity, eager to descend ninety steps below street level to enter the "Empire of Death," otherwise known as the Paris Catacombs. In this new space, which opened to the public in 1809, visitors passed through a series of tunnels and caverns that were lined from floor to ceiling with carefully stacked and arranged human bones. Although each section of the Catacombs featured distinctive components, such as a lacrimatory vase, a small pond of goldfish, or a sepulchral lamp, most of the underground tour would have featured the same view of unidentifiable and indistinguishable human remains (figure 4.1). As Etienne de Jouy, publishing as the Hermit of the Chausée-d'Antin, described the site in 1812:

Bones bend into arcs [and] rise into columns, an artistic hand created a kind of mosaic out of these final remains of humanity, whose ordered regularity only adds to the profound contemplation that this space inspires. . . . Ten generations have been swallowed up here, and this subterranean population is estimated to be three times larger than its aboveground counterpart. . . . Inscriptions, placed on limestone pillars, indicate which Parisian neighborhoods once contained these remains. Here, all distinctions of sex, wealth, and rank have finally disappeared.[1]

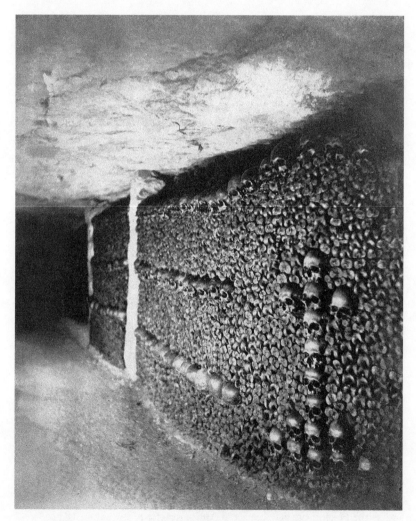

Figure 4.1. Nadar [Gaspard Félix Tournachon], *The Catacombs of Paris. The Final Gallery*, 1861. The J. Paul Getty Museum. Digital Image courtesy of the Getty's Open Content Program.

Like Père Lachaise, the Catacombs made space for the dead and provided interested Parisians, like Jouy, with the opportunity to reimagine their postrevolutionary city. By surrounding himself with "ten generations" of his anonymous and indistinguishable predecessors, Jouy experienced a version of his city in which crucial social distinctions had "finally" given way to quiet harmony.

Although they share a similar timeline and were both exemplars of the new Parisian burial culture, Père Lachaise Cemetery and the Paris Catacombs contrasted severely with one another, throwing each other's innovations into sharp relief. Père Lachaise was located on a hill overlooking the city, while the Catacombs were deep under the ground; the cemetery exalted and celebrated the dead as individuals, while the Catacombs only displayed them en masse; Père Lachaise accommodated and accented the divide between the wealthy and the poor in the city, while the Catacombs revealed the fleeting nature of such difference. Accordingly, some of Père Lachaise's fiercest champions, men like François-Marie Marchant de Beaumont, were among the Catacombs' chief detractors. In contrast to Jouy's admiration, Marchant de Beaumont critiqued the new ossuary precisely because of the anonymity and uniformity of the bones on display. He hated that the bones of so many illustrious Parisians were commingling with—and indistinguishable from—the remains of "vulgar men." After a few minutes underground, to highlight his contempt for the Catacombs' democratic aesthetic, Marchant de Beaumont began tapping his fingers on the skulls out of idle curiosity.[2]

The differences between Jouy and Marchant de Beaumont also played out among the many ordinary Parisians who visited the Catacombs and responded to the site's unique ability to obliterate difference and emphasize commonality across boundaries of class, gender, and history. Many saw a reflection of themselves in the façade, such as an 1811 visitor who wrote of the bones: "They were what I am, and I will be what they are." For others, descending underground was a profoundly religious experience that recalled the fundamental equality of all souls before God: "Death imparts a terrifying uniformity to its subjects: power, talent, and beauty are all mixed together. God alone knows how to distinguish virtues." As with twenty-first-century crowds, however, not everyone took the space so seriously, choosing instead to interpret the Catacombs as an amusing and thrilling way to spend an afternoon, or a "beautiful horror" as one 1812 guest exclaimed.[3]

While such a broad set of interpretations and reactions makes it difficult to generalize about the meaning of the Catacombs, this resistance to easy categorization also provides valuable insight into how the Catacombs functioned in the postrevolutionary city. At a time when the state and population were attempting to understand (or forget) and consolidate (or move beyond) the tumult of the revolutionary decade, the Catacombs offered a safe and stable venue for this difficult work. The built environment of the Catacombs was essential to its power because while they remained intimately connected to the city through their skeletal contents, the Catacombs were at a significant remove from the aboveground world. This separation was both conceptual—as the "Empire of Death"—and physical, since the ossuary's liminal location, at the city's edge and below its streets, amplified this distance. Additionally, while they retained a thrilling illusion of danger, the Catacombs were the public face (or, perhaps, its skull) of a state engineering project to stabilize the capital from the (under)ground up.

It took decades for the French state to create a functioning ossuary out of an ancient quarry. What began as an expedient solution to the storage problem posed by the closing of the Cemetery of the Innocents became by the early nineteenth century a sensational public monument with not-so-subtle ties to the problematic legacy of the French Revolution. However, the state lost control of this strange new monument as soon as they opened it up to the public, between 1809 and 1830. As the samples that opened this chapter hint, despite the uniformity of the bones on display, the Paris Catacombs almost immediately proved itself to be capable of sustaining a range of meanings for its postrevolutionary audience. In its earliest incarnation the Catacombs developed into an unexpectedly inclusive space where Parisians of all ideological persuasions could air their anxieties about the present and their hopes for the future.

Understanding the ways in which early visitors inscribed a range of (often conflicting) meanings onto the Catacombs is difficult because of a paucity of source materials. However, this chapter relies heavily on a historically underused manuscript: the Catacombs' guestbook. This *Registre des visiteurs* covers the period from July 1809 until August 1813 and contains a remarkable range of viewpoints from both female and male visitors of all ages and from a variety of backgrounds. Although most of the individuals who filled the book with extended comments were relatively educated men, Catacombs visitors actually represented a wide range of the population from Paris, France, and Europe. As a source, the guestbook can be problematic, since it is by its very nature anecdotal and resistant to any single narrative. As an 1830 article in the *Revue des deux mondes* noted, the contents of the guestbook were simultaneously profound, bizarre, and curious.[4] However, when read alongside contemporary published descriptions, the guestbook's many voices provide valuable insight into the range of possible reactions, interpretations, and concerns among the Catacombs' first generation of visitors.

From Quarry to Catacomb

When he visited the Paris Catacombs a decade after they opened to the public, John Griscom, an American travel writer, described them as "subterranean wonders" and "cavernous passages in the limestone strata, on which the city of Paris is founded."[5] The Catacombs had many physical and imagined features that accented this powerful image of the ossuary as a foundation for the capital. The most fundamental of these was intimately bound up in its origin story, in which a neglected network of subterranean tunnels was transformed from an imminent threat into a solid base between the 1770s and the first decade of the nineteenth century.

For centuries subterranean Paris had been associated with a whole range of fears and anxieties about crime and danger. Since the thirteenth century, the underground quarries had sheltered smugglers, vagabonds, and various malefactors, including by some accounts the devil himself. In the seventeenth century, a clever entrepreneur known simply as César exploited this infernal association by selling tickets into the devil's subterranean Parisian lair—César was later imprisoned for his antics and died in the Bastille in 1615.[6] Similarly, throughout the eighteenth century, the tunnels beneath Paris were reputed to harbor dangerous and socially undesirable types, including Jean-Paul Marat, who may have caught his famous skin disease from spending too much time underground. As late as 1801, the Préfecture de Police cautioned city dwellers to block off any access to the underground from their basements, lest they become a dangerous "haven for criminals."[7]

In addition to these persistent criminal associations, by the last quarter of the eighteenth century the subterranean world endangered the living much more tangibly, by threatening to crack open and engulf the city into its murky caverns. Since antiquity, Parisians had been mining their underground to extract necessary building materials, most notably limestone. Initially, these excavations had taken place outside of the urban center, but over the centuries the city expanded over the once-peripheral subterranean system of mines and tunnels. As Paris grew from the fourteenth to the eighteenth century, the state seemingly forgot its predecessors' caution, and increased excavation activity to meet the demands of construction. In the early nineteenth century, a Jacobin-turned-guidebook-author, Jacques-Antoine Dulaure, interpreted this rapacious hollowing out of the capital as evidence of Bourbon France's irresponsible and inept administration. As he recounted it, the government's indifference, ignorance, and non-existent supervision had placed in peril large parts of the city. Important urban landmarks, including the Observatory, Luxembourg Palace, and the Panthéon, he explained, were all "founded on the emptiness of the immense quarries" and "suspended over an abyss."[8]

This threatening "abyss" became especially evident in the 1770s when streets in the southeastern corner of the city began breaking down and opening up. Most infamously, an eighty-four-foot sinkhole appeared in the rue d'Enfer near the Saint-Michel barrier in 1774.[9] Four years later, a collapse in Menilmontant swallowed up seven people, some of whose bodies were later recovered eighty feet below street level.[10] After these collapses became more regular and the population grew increasingly nervous about the stability of their property, the government ordered a small contingent of architects and police to inspect the quarries for safety. This soon grew into a permanent commission, and shortly thereafter the Ministry of the Interior created the Service des carrières to map, reinforce, and permanently maintain the underground system of tunnels. A famous Parisian architect, Charles-Axel Guillaumon, was named inspector general of the quarries with a mandate to ensure that no more houses (or people) sank into the earth.[11]

This new attention to the Parisian underground ultimately paved the way for the creation of the municipal ossuary. When the Cemetery of the Innocents was closed down in 1780, the recently mapped and reinforced network of tunnels provided an ideal storage solution for the eight centuries' worth of human bones that were about to be disinterred.

Marc Viré has noted that during this time, the idea of a Parisian Catacombs was discussed fairly regularly among those concerned.[12] For example, in 1782, an anonymous author who published under the name
"Villedieu" wrote a short essay that commended Paris's good fortune, because "the hand of art, driven by that of chance" had "perfectly prepared"
a "catacomb" for the city's dead.[13] Four years later a modified version of
this project was put into practice, and on the evening of April 7, 1786, a
small group of clergymen and administrators gathered to consecrate the
Paris Catacombs. From that point forward, regular nighttime cortèges to
the Catacombs transported cartloads of human bones into jumbled piles
underground. These transfers continued throughout the early years of the
Revolution before coming to an abrupt (and temporary) end in 1793.

The Catacombs sat unused and relatively forgotten for over a decade
after the Terror. As one contemporary article put it, "During the succes-
sive revolutions which distracted France, the Catacombs fell into a state
of confusion, and in many places, of ruin; the air had become stagnant
and unwholesome, and water, oozing from above, had rendered them extremely unsafe."[14] Government documents from the second half of the
1790s support these rumors of dilapidation. Although the Service des carrières oversaw annual inspections and ongoing projects to stabilize and
reinforce the underground, terrain was constantly collapsing throughout
Paris. Beginning in 1795, individuals from the Department of Civic Buildings and the Ministry of the Interior all implored the newly elected Executive Directory to allocate an annual fund for the maintenance of the
Parisian underground. In increasingly urgent tones, they argued that while
things had improved since the 1770s, the underground became less stable
every day, as it threatened to "spontaneously" crack open and "swallow
up" citizens.[15] The Minister of the Interior exclaimed that "all that was
most precious in the Republic" lay suspended over an abyss and warned
that many parts of the department of the Seine were in serious danger of
being engulfed in the "entrails of the earth."[16]

The executive of the Directory turned down the request for a regular bud-
get dedicated to the maintenance of the underground, but it did so without
necessarily refusing the funds. In a move that revealed much about popular sensitivity on this issue, they requested that as much money as necessary be directed at this problem, provided that the whole situation was kept
quiet. Concerned that the weakness of the city's foundation might terrify

both the legislative body and the citizens of Paris, the Executive Directory made clear that these operations needed to take place with the "utmost secrecy."[17] Throughout the latter half of the 1790s and the beginning of the nineteenth century, reports continued to flood in about various sink-holes throughout the city. Early in 1802, three small holes appeared in a garden belonging to Citizen Boulard on rue Faubourg Saint-Marcel. The Service des carrières promptly visited the quarries underneath the entire quarter and urged local inhabitants to keep their distance from the garden. Shortly after taking these precautions, a new hole, this time ten meters in diameter and seven meters deep appeared. The service successfully repaired the problem, but one can hardly imagine that it remained secret for very long.[18]

Within a few years the situation seems to have come under control, and in March 1809 the minister of the interior injected the Service des carrières with new life by appointing a thirty-three-year-old engineer, Louis-Étienne Héricart de Thury, to a position of leadership in the department of mines and quarries. One of Héricart de Thury's first orders of business was to substantially renovate the municipal ossuary and transform it from a repository of scattered bones into a public monument. Within four months enough work had been completed to open the space up to the public.

The Miserable Bones

Between 1786 and 1808, the Catacombs grew increasingly full of human bones, but they did not take on their now-famous appearance until 1809. As Héricart de Thury and his staff worked to convert the ossuary into a public monument they transformed its aesthetic from hasty piles of bones into careful stacks and artful structures. Héricart de Thury, a meticulous engineer, deemed it necessary to transform the Catacombs from barely contained chaos to ordered regularity. "I believed it was necessary to take special care in the conservation of this monument," he explained on the eve of the Catacombs' grand opening, "considering the intimate rapport that will surely exist between the Catacombs and the events of the French Revolution." To accomplish this task, "the interior was restored, the ventilation system was improved, bones were arranged with as much art as skill. Nothing was spared to make this monument worthy of public veneration."[19]

By mentioning the "events" of the Revolution, Héricart de Thury invoked the fact that in addition to millions of bones from closed Parisian cemeteries, the Catacombs harbored a much more controversial collection of human remains that were the unhappy result of some of the Revolution's most infamous *journées*. Although the Catacombs usually behaved as a secondary burial site, similar to a charnel house, on several occasions during the early Revolution they became an expedient primary burial site. After royal guards shot and killed several Parisians during a celebration in August 1788, they transported their bodies directly to the Catacombs. The Réveillon Riots a year later saw several more people buried immediately in the Catacombs after falling to royal bullets. Most notoriously, as many as a thousand prisoners from the 1792 September Massacres found their way underground following the bloody days.[20] In each of these instances, the Catacombs served as a useful space where problematic corpses could be quickly stashed away in anonymity and forgotten, since the Catacombs were not yet an accessible city space.

Héricart de Thury's "events" of the Revolution seems a clear reference to these violent episodes. Yet, does this imply a counterrevolutionary expiatory intent or simply a commemorative one? Héricart de Thury's biography offers some answers. Although he came of age under the First Republic and achieved professional success during the Empire, he was from a noble family that dated its privilege back to the fifteenth century. After the Restoration, Héricart de Thury was recognized for his loyalty and devotion to the Monarchy. In his acclaimed and widely read description of the Catacombs (published in 1815), he noted that what made the Paris Catacombs particularly unique was their ability to "honor the reign of the best of kings, and the most unfortunate Monarch, Louis XVI."[21] He was also one of the very few people in France who was wealthy enough to be elected to the Chamber of Deputies in 1815, where he sat with the ultraroyalist faction. His recent biographers refer to Héricart de Thury unambiguously as a resolute royalist and a "very pious and deeply faithful" Catholic.[22] In 1814, he even erected a small expiatory altar in front of the September bones, which he had previously concealed from view by a painted black wall.[23]

The bones from the September Massacres became a mainstay in published descriptions of the Catacombs, which began appearing after 1812. Almost immediately it became something of a cliché for authors to write about people (usually young women) swooning in front of these frightening

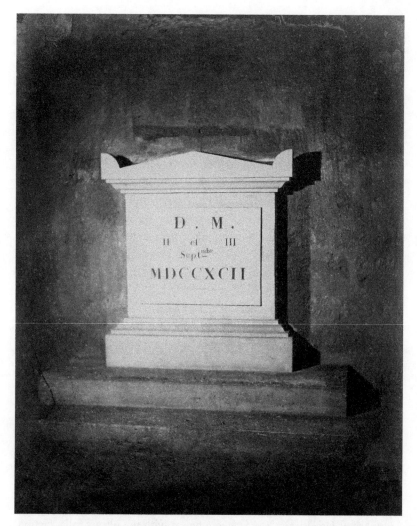

Figure 4.2. Nadar [Gaspard Félix Tournachon], *The Catacombs of Paris, Cippe commemoratif des 2 et 3 septembre 1792*, 1861. The J. Paul Getty Museum. Digital Image courtesy of the Getty's Open Content Program.

reminders of revolutionary violence. In the *Gazette de France* Etienne de Jouy described the September bones as "more horrifying" than the rest of the space and noted that the young woman who accompanied him on his visit let out a "cry of horror" when she thought she heard a low moan emanating from the sad remains.[24] An English article, closely modeled after Jouy's similarly referred to a "sylph-like" French woman who "sank into the arms of her deeply affected husband, who kissed the pearly drops from her silken lashes" when she imagined that the "ashes of her murdered parents" were among the September bones.[25] As an arresting visual and physical reminder of one of the Revolution's most infamous moments, these bones were also a particularly important pilgrimage site for conservative visitors. When the duc d'Angoulême (the son of the future Charles X) toured the Catacombs privately with Héricart de Thury in 1818, he was especially moved by "the burial that was secretly given to the miserable victims of the prison massacres and other events of our Revolution."[26] In Abbé Guillon's 1821 *Martyrologie* of the Revolution, he claimed that the expiatory altar attracted "an infinite amount of people motivated by piety or compassion" to the Catacombs.[27]

Outside of published descriptions, however, the small monument to the September Massacres does not seem to have made a substantial impact. The guestbook that Héricart de Thury placed at the Catacombs' exit contains fewer than ten comments that explicitly reference the Revolution, and even fewer that mention the September Massacres. Since thousands of individuals inscribed the book between 1809 and 1813, this absence is notable. Those who did invoke violence stand out, such as "Professeur Celebrini," who transcribed two short J. B. Rousseau poems and dedicated one of them to the remains of the victims of the September Massacres. Similarly, on August 6, 1812, "Dupont" wrote that his heart was frozen with horror and cried out for the victims of the Terror. Several days later someone else composed a poem that described the bones as the victims of wicked men that would forever "attest to the evils of our Republic."[28] These passages are evocative and well-composed, but they are also exceptional and represent only a minuscule fraction of Catacombs visitors; most either missed, ignored, or defied Héricart de Thury's expiatory intent. For example, a group of French soldiers who visited in 1813 wrote that after their underground tour they were inspired to feel "honor and love of the fatherland." However, ten days later, C. Crouserieu inscribed the book by predicting that if a perpetrator of the September Massacres ever made his way underground, he would surely tremble with remorse.[29] On the most banal level this meant that one person's expiatory space could be another's patriotic monument, but it also indicates how mutable the Catacombs could be. As a site that spoke in different voices to different audiences, the Catacombs were remarkably adept at navigating both sides of 1789. Despite Héricart de Thury's hope that the Catacombs might serve as a somber memorial to the victims of revolutionary violence, he lost control of the ossuary's meaning as soon as he opened its doors to the curious public.

The Beautiful Horror of the Catacombs

On a visit to Paris in the summer of 1816, the English antiquary Seth William Stevenson complained that in the Catacombs, "the horror-struck countenances of some were opposed to the ill-timed frivolity of gesture and discourse indulged in by others."[30] Similarly, another individual, filled a half-page of the Catacombs' guestbook on April 24, 1811, with complaints about those who visited the Catacombs out of curiosity, lacked respect for their fellow men, and even showed contempt for the bones they came across.[31] Both of these critics observed a phenomenon that has characterized the Catacombs for more than two hundred years. Almost since the moment that they opened to the public, the Catacombs have been a source of fascination, curiosity, and amusement. In the second half of the nineteenth century, they provided the backdrop for several horror stories.[32] More recently, the Catacombs have appeared in Hollywood movies, a French series of graphic novels, and feature stories in *National Geographic* and *Smithsonian* magazine online.[33] Critics like Stevenson remind us that this tendency to treat the Catacombs as an entertaining lark has always been integral to their appeal, for better or for worse. One early visitor recorded feeling "joy and pleasure" during his tour of the Catacombs and many others wrote strangely lighthearted comments such as: "I've seen death, it is in front of my eyes, but my stomach is grumbling, and I'd much rather eat."[34] Several visitors also made a point of explaining how the Catacombs had made them laugh or smile. Jacques-Antoine Dulaure, commented on this phenomenon in one of his books, noting that the Catacombs' guestbook was filled with "so much silliness."[35]

Early nineteenth-century visitors to the Catacombs interpreted this lighthearted approach to the Catacombs as altogether new, distinctively Parisian, and deeply concerning. For example, someone calling himself the "Solitaire du marais" inveighed against "All of Paris, Paris corrupted / Who gaily visits tombs / and laughs again at the catacombs."[36] Pierre-François Piétresson de Saint-Aubin similarly described the guestbook comments as singsong inscriptions that almost all belonged to disturbingly frivolous Parisians.[37] And an 1830 article that compared Irish to French Catacombs noted that the main difference between the two was that in the Paris Catacombs, "a fantastic and artificial combination make light of death; it is melodrama imported into the nether regions. How I shudder to think of the somber gravity of eternity mingling with this superficial display of bones and skeletons!" The author concluded: "A fondness for pretty things must be so powerful in Paris to have penetrated all the way to its catacombs."[38] This critic invoked the familiar trope of indecent, frivolous postrevolutionary Parisians, but his allusion to popular fiction warrants further analysis because it invokes a much bigger cultural phenomenon of the period in which fear and entertainment were inexorably intertwined.

At the turn of the nineteenth century, Parisians displayed an increased fascination with the macabre, terrifying, and sublime that extended well beyond the Catacombs. Wax displays had been popular in the city since the 1770s, but after the Revolution broke out, entrepreneurs such as Philippe Curtius and his adopted niece Marie Tussaud began displaying grisly scenes of guillotined heads and simulations of death.[39] The late eighteenth century also witnessed the rise of Fantasmagoria: theatrical demonstrations that promised to reveal ghostly apparitions—including the ghosts of Jean-Paul Marat and Robespierre—to paying visitors.[40] Perhaps the best-known features of the postrevolutionary cult of the macabre are the horror stories and Gothic novels that became extremely popular in France at the turn of the nineteenth century. In his 1800 work on the novel the Marquis de Sade offered the most famous explanation for the popularity of the macabre after the French Revolution, arguing that after the public bloodshed and mass killings of the 1790s, contemporary writers had no other recourse than to think up even more horrifying scenarios to entertain audiences.[41] De Sade's theory overstates how desensitized to violence the French population had become, but it usefully reiterates how prevalent these themes were in postrevolutionary popular culture. In the early nineteenth century, Parisians enjoyed being scared.

In its visual presentation, the Catacombs had many things in common with the macabre culture of its period. Like the settings of Gothic novels, the Catacombs offered access to an ambiguously "old" space filled with historical secrets, created a strong sense of the uncanny through its prominently featured skulls, and invoked an unmistakable sense of liminality that united opposites like life/death and above/below. Owing to its labyrinthine structure, gloomy decor, and association with death and destruction, it is entirely possible that the Catacombs may have seemed like a real-life Gothic adventure to those who ventured underground. Moreover, as with fantasmagamoric shows and wax museums, the Catacombs participated in the cultural phenomenon of seeking pleasure from simulations of what had recently been very real threats. To this end, the Catacombs presented the dead in a securely constructed space that nonetheless recalled danger and destruction.

By 1809 the transition from abandoned quarry to stylized ossuary unburdened the underground from any actual danger, but many still felt as though they were taking their life into their own hands when they descended the Empire of Death. When eager visitors gathered at the Catacombs' entrance, their tour guide sternly warned them *never* to deviate from the group, lest they fall behind, take a wrong turn, and get lost in the dark abyss. "The most imminent danger would attend a separation of the visitor from their guide," wrote an American tourist and travel writer in 1823. "A black line is drawn upon the wall of the principal avenue, but this clue might be insufficient to lead the stranger to the regions of day-light and courage would fail him,—his taper become extinguished,—and death in its most appalling form, overwhelm him."[42] Nestor Lamarque similarly imagined the terrifying prospect of being trapped in the Catacombs, fatally out of sight and earshot from the world above ground.[43] An image from a bilingual 1823 book of "picturesque views of the city of Paris and its environs" reiterates this aura of danger and subtly references the underground's historic instability: skulls tumble around a male visitor who seems to have wandered away from his group, finding himself alone in a dark cavern with skulls at his feet and crumbling pillars around him (fig 4.3).

The Catacombs also "threatened" their visitors by bringing them into close proximity with the very contents that had caused so much distress at the end of the eighteenth century when the dead had laid in decrepit urban churchyards. Once they were underground, the former residents of the Cemetery of the Innocents were stripped of their bodies and consequently their infectious miasmas. As one visitor succinctly wrote in the guestbook, "why be afraid [?] the dead can't hurt you."[44] Yet, with a little bit of imagination, some visitors to the Catacombs could still evoke the

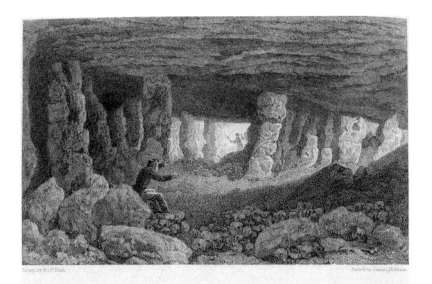

THE CATACOMBS.

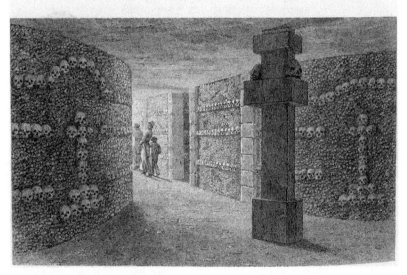

Figure 4.3. Frederick Nash, "The Paris Catacombs," *Picturesque Views of the City of Paris and Its Environs* (London, 1823). The Newberry Library, Chicago (folio G 397.802).

dead as a threat, albeit psychological rather than physiological. At the end of his published description of the Catacombs in 1816, Pierre-François Piétresson de Saint-Aubin addressed any readers who might visit the Catacombs out of curiosity and without any strong emotional response to the "frightening heaps of debris from past generations." He warned them that about halfway through their visit, their blasé affect would break down as they began to feel overwhelmed by the death that surrounded them. As Piétresson de Saint-Aubin elaborated: "A secret horror seizes you, you flee . . . but in vain; the terrible spectacle of the Catacombs accompanies you, it pursues you, and for days you see nothing in front of you but hideous skeletons who seem jealous of your existence and endeavor to tear it from you."[45]

Piétresson de Saint-Aubin's jealous skeletons seem to be an aggressive and graphic memento mori: the author's attempt to extract meaning from the bones for his readers, much as he did when describing Père Lachaise Cemetery. But by framing his advice in the language of the macabre, he invoked nineteenth-century trends in popular culture. This connection to the fantastic did more than attract visitors; it reinforced the Catacombs' capacity to act as a theater for anxieties about the problems of postrevolutionary society more broadly. As many scholars, including Peter Brooks, Ronald Schechter, and José Monléon have remarked, recourse to terrifying narratives in the early nineteenth century was intimately bound up in the perceived social and moral instability of the new era, which Brooks evocatively describes as "a frightening new world in which the traditional patterns of moral order no longer provide the necessary social glue."[46] By constructing literary worlds filled with characters that faced the looming threat of moral chaos, authors could satisfy their readers with happy endings in which the good and virtuous emerged triumphant. Similarly, touring the Catacombs provided Parisians with the opportunity to temporarily (and safely) surround themselves with death and the illusion of danger. Moreover, the "scary" and carnivalesque atmosphere of the Catacombs provided an unlikely refuge from an aboveground world in a seemingly constant state of change.

The Confused Equality of Death

To contemporaries reflecting on the postrevolutionary condition of France, one of the most distinctive characteristics of Parisian society was a remarkable sense of flux: the traditional social order had not survived the Revolution, but nothing new appeared to have replaced it. As an English visitor to Paris described it in 1815: "The self-respect which keeps each class distinct in our country, yet does not *seek* occasion to show itself, seems here unknown. All degrees in society appear mixt together and confounded like a shuffled pack of cards, and will require a considerable time to be sorted and re-arranged."[47] The Catacombs, with its masses of similar and unidentifiable bones, offered a stark visual analog to a postrevolutionary social scenario, which could seem either exhilarating or threatening of looming social chaos, depending on one's perspective. Several decades later, the Catacombs' famous first photographer, Nadar, summed up these sentiments when he evocatively referred to the Catacombs' arrangement as "this confused equality of death."[48] Thomas Détruisard, a curate from Gentilly who published one of the earliest descriptions of the Catacombs in 1812, referred to the Catacombs in similar tones, judging them alternately "terrible" and "instructive." He also imagined what it might look like "if all the people who once belonged to these inanimate remains" suddenly woke up, reassembled themselves and appeared before him. "We would see, alas! what we cannot avoid," he explained, "that virtue is mixed up with crime, opulence with misery, good sense with foolishness, brilliance with stupidity, wisdom with folly . . . *and finally, humility with pride and modesty with presumption.*[49] Détruisard's discomfort with the organization of the bones reflected two related concerns that plagued France after the end of the Terror in 1794: the reconstruction of social morality (moeurs) without the structure of the Catholic Church, and the problematic application of equality in France. These concerns would persist throughout the nineteenth century but were particularly salient in the early nineteenth century, because they concerned the difficulty of understanding and implementing the goals of the French Revolution without reigniting domestic violence, strife, and instability. The Catacombs became an unconventional but useful venue where the population could temporarily resolve these problems.

For many who toured the Catacombs, the anonymity and uniformity of the bones on display was a powerful reminder that "everyone is equal here." One visitor noted on October 15, 1810, that he and his companions had tried but failed to distinguish the bones of the rich from those of the poor. On December 26 of the following year, another wrote that in the Catacombs, "the nobleman is nothing but a pile of dust." Many others made similar, but simpler comments, pointing out that "equality, constant equality, here you take back your rights" or "true Equality is here." Taking a more confrontational tone, Louis Soehnée, who visited the Catacombs three times in May 1812, challenged "all of you petty squabblers" to "argue over the primitive equality of men!"[50] In 1815 Léon Thiessé published a poem about the Catacombs, a great "depot of death" where "the greatest of enemies" all slumbered together and became friends.[51] Similarly, in a published 1812 article, the Hermit of Saint-Germain (M. Colnet) compared the Catacombs to aboveground Parisian cemeteries where the wealthy could still "buy the right to decay" in isolation from the poor. Underground, there were "no more monuments, no more epitaphs, no more brilliant deceptions: oblivion is naked, one sees nothing but bones." Colnet continued by noting that only the Catacombs could reunite "the most bitter enemies," like Jesuits and Jansenists, who spent their whole lives arguing without ever actually hearing one another. "Go ahead and argue, my good friends," he concluded. "This is what it has taken to force you to be quiet and come together."[52]

Colnet's jeer was clearly meant to ridicule the futility of French Catholic factionalism, but such comments, which reveled in the leveling effect of death, also drew on old habits of interpreting death as the great equalizer. In this sense, the "primitive equality" of the bones on display was itself open to various interpretations. Indeed, Thomas Détruisard's anxious comment in which he imagined the resurrection of the Catacombs was undoubtedly informed by his own Catholicism. Many visitors inscribed the guestbook with passages from much older poems in the Catholic tradition of memento mori. For example, François de Malherbe's 1592 work "Consolation à M. Du Perier sur la mort de sa fille" was quoted at least a dozen times by particularly literate visitors. This poem warned that "Death has his rigorous laws. . . . The poor man in his hut, with only thatch for cover, Unto these laws must bend, The sentinel that guards the barriers of the Louvre Cannot our kings defend."[53] The possible implications of the persistence of this tradition is striking, particularly since the purpose of memento mori was ostensibly not only to remind the audience of their mortality, but to shock them into a more observant lifestyle. In both published descriptions and the guestbook comments, ample evidence exists to suggest that many Parisians did indeed interpret the Catacombs as a religious (Christian) space. For example, in May 1811 one guest wrote that "one hour in the Catacombs is worth a year of sermons," while others were inspired to consoling religious thoughts, such as "one look to the heavens assuages my pain" or "what a terrible, but consoling spectacle for the religious man."[54]

The assortment of placards that adorned the walls of the Catacombs further enhanced (and complicated) the underground monument's "religious" tone. In 1810, after the Catacombs had been opened to the public for about a year, Héricart de Thury decided to erect a set of small signs throughout the ossuary inscribed with inspirational maxims about death culled from a wide range of sources, including the Bible, Stoics such as Marcus Aurelius and Seneca, and more recent French poets like Lafontaine, Legouvé, and Delille. This eclectic collection was very much a product of its time, reflecting Napoleonic religious policy and culture. As Jacques-Olivier Boudon has demonstrated, Napoleon was equally committed to preserving the power of a Catholic Church (albeit under state control) and respecting the Enlightenment commitment to religious pluralism.[55] In truth, Héricart de Thury was probably not entirely on board with this aspect of the Catacombs' aesthetic—his original list was subjected to state censorship—but in his 1815 published description of the Catacombs, he was fairly clear about the message he was hoping to craft. He admitted that as a devout Catholic, he found the (ir)religious implications of many ancient texts troubling, so he flanked them with inscriptions that confirmed the existence of a Christian afterlife.[56]

Most published descriptions of the placards were critical, complaining of the "incongruous mixture of opposite sentiments" and admonishing Héricart de Thury for allowing "the false philosophy" of "the Encyclopedists" to "mingle" with more conventional inscriptions of memento mori.[57] Etienne de Jouy similarly disapproved of "this mixture of contradictory opinions," and in 1815 the English travel writer John Scott concluded: "Nothing could be more gloomy to the mind, or more unsuitable to the nature of the place than this confusion of creeds."[58] Yet the guests who inscribed the guestbook responded much more positively to the ambiguously religious tone of the space. One entry urged "men of the world, philosophers of all sects, politicians of all countries," to look on the Catacombs and meditate.[59] Many more referred to feeling a generally "religious respect" or having "religious thoughts" for a space so "religiously executed."[60] One visitor from May 1812 characterized the Catacombs as one of the most imposing, but religious, monuments that s/he had ever seen.[61] Virtually no one inscribing the guestbook admonished Héricart de Thury or critiqued his aesthetic. Several explicitly thanked him for his industriousness, good taste, and sensibility.[62]

The most commonly expressed sentiment in the guestbook was also the most banal: "here, one can learn how to live."[63] Dozens of inscriptions contained some version of this very basic tenet of memento mori that encouraged the living to improve their lives by contemplating their own impending death. Yet, as art historian Suzanne Lindsay recently argued, the eighteenth century in France witnessed the advent of a modified memento mori, in which the omnipresence of corpses in public view provided opportunities to mediate new concerns.[64] While it is very likely that certain Catacombs tourists emerged from their subterranean visit with renewed or strengthened faith, it seems just as possible that they would be inclined to contemplate recently politicized ideas such as equality or religious pluralism and toleration. The unusual visual presentation of the Catacombs provided guests with the opportunity to see the space through either (or both) of these lenses.

The Story of the Past, Present, and Future

The anonymity of the bones in the Catacombs imbued the underground with a kind of ideological malleability that accommodated different—and often contrasting—meanings to an audience that was alternately Catholic, agnostic, republican, and royalist. This capacity to hold in balance so many postrevolutionary voices ultimately created a space where visitors could navigate thorny revolutionary legacies and lingering debates over the place of religion and the meaning of equality in the early nineteenth century. As many historians have already shown, this process of accommodation, in which revolutionary projects and ideology combined with quotidian realities, was the direct result of a much bigger and broader search for order after the Revolution. Between 1786 when the Catacombs were first inaugurated and 1809, when they opened to the public, Parisians experienced five forms of government, thousands of public deaths, and fifteen years (and counting) of war. On a more mundane level, street names periodically changed, neologisms took on epic proportions, and the state adopted an entirely new method of measuring time between 1793 and 1805. The direct effect of this rapid, extreme, and near-constant change was a keen desire for stability, which manifested as a range of new practices that ultimately shaped modern French political and social identity. Suzanne Desan, Jennifer Heuer, and Denise Davidson have convincingly demonstrated the gendered dimension of this phenomenon, calling attention to postrevolutionary policies and practices that were designed to stabilize the social order and provide a secure route to national belonging through hierarchical family structures.[65] Similarly, James Livesey, Isser Woloch, Andrew Jainchill, and others have illustrated the long-term political consequences of the postrevolutionary condition.[66]

The early history of the Catacombs illuminates a different, but equally crucial process of accommodation, in which Parisians sought a soothing remedy for the Revolution's much-vaunted historical break. Many scholars have commented on the growing discontinuity between the past and the present around the turn of the nineteenth century, from Foucault's "irruptive violence of time" to Peter Fritzsche's "melancholy of history."[67] It is similarly well known that the early nineteenth century in Europe was consequently characterized by a newfound fascination with the past. Stephen Bann has gone so far as to claim that this intense "desire for history" was one of the defining features of the Romantic era.[68] In this climate of historical instability and longing, the Catacombs—filled with "ten generations" of Parisians—offered unprecedented and tangible access to a past that had grown increasingly remote since the radical historical break of 1789 divided "old" from "new."

Many early nineteenth-century authors remarked on the relationship between Paris and its Catacombs in terms that evoked an intimate urban history. An anonymously published poem about visiting the Catacombs on the Day of the Dead described the entrance to the Catacombs as a deep and plunging chasm that transported visitors into the city's "bosom" and brought them into contact with past centuries, assembled in the abyss.[69] Significantly, these were not Victor Hugo's "intestines of leviathan," the notorious sewers beneath Paris that acted as the city's conscience and repository for all its dirty secrets. Instead, the Catacombs provided a structurally and historically supportive framework for Paris, what Héricart de Thury described as the city's "lining." The Catacombs' rapport with the history of Paris was immediately evident to every visitor because each section of displayed bones was accompanied by an identifying label that indicated their cemetery of origin and the year of their transfer underground. Early tourists would have known, for example, whether they were standing in front of the "Bones from the Cemetery of the Innocents deposited in April 1786" or the "Bones from the cemetery of St. Landry [deposited on] June 18, 1792."[70] These simple markers clarified how the aboveground city mapped onto its underground, as they reconstructed a revolutionary migration of the dead, in which ten generations of bones had been relocated into a new "bizarre city."[71]

An unconventional narrative of Parisian history also played out in two small, but meticulously arranged displays that Héricart de Thury organized for public view with the help of M. Gambier Lapierre, the keeper of the Catacombs. The first was a mineralogical collection, which included every kind of soil and rock from the earth beneath the city as well as some fossils, shells, and pieces of an ancient Roman aqueduct. A second "pathological" collection displayed deformed, diseased, and decomposing bones (mostly culled from the Cemetery of the Innocents), which Héricart de Thury set up so that visitors could witness "with a single glance, all traces and degrees in the slow march of destruction."[72] Both collections emphasized the natural history contained in the Catacombs while also highlighting the ongoing geological and biological processes that were perpetually at work. As the head engineer for Paris's mines and quarries, Héricart de Thury was particularly interested in finding meaning and significance in the city's underground. His displays reflect an early nineteenth-century penchant for archaeology and a desire to interpret the subterranean world as a potentially rich source of historical knowledge.[73]

The most obvious "historical" feature of the Catacombs was, of course, the "Bona fide debris of our fathers."[74] Much like the slow march of destruction and change on display, some visitors also read the anonymous bones as evidence of another never-ending cycle—one that told "the story of the past, the present, and the future," as one guest described it.[75] On January 23, 1809, a man named Guillaume who worked for the department of tax collection visited the Catacombs and concisely described the phenomenon that linked these populations to each other and to their city: "Throughout their lives they worked the earth. After their lives, their bodies support that same earth."[76] Thomas Détruisard's published essay on the Catacombs made a similar observation about the organic reversal that took place under Paris's streets. In 1812 he contemplated how "these two million individuals, who for centuries made up part of the population of this immense city, have now . . . replaced the material that once harbored them, and now harbor those who will soon join them in death."[77] M. Gouriet's 1816 poem about the Catacombs made a similar—though much grimmer—observation about "the ravages of time" at work underground and expressed no small amount of horror at the "numberless generations" that were "swallowed up" by the "immense ruin" of the Catacombs. "Paris! Oh Paris" he asked, distraught and trembling, "is that you?"[78] As though answering Gouriet's appeal, one Catacombs visitor from July 1812 inscribed the guestbook by writing: "It's Paris returned!"[79]

An 1812 visitor to the Catacombs urged Parisians to "cherish this space because it contains the bones of your forefathers."[80] The guestbook provides many examples of individuals who followed this advice, such as Laure Desfontaines who wrote "pleased to see you all again" after her tour.[81] Guests hoping to feel reunited with specific individuals were usually disappointed; one woman lamented that despite passing through the entire collection, she was unable to recognize her husband's remains.[82] The thoroughly unimpressed François-Marie Marchant de Beaumont similarly criticized the Catacombs for rendering previous illustrious Parisians anonymous: "They were our family, our friends, our elders; their talents, their piety, their wisdom exemplified our patrie; they enriched it with their work or defended it through their courage."[83] Yet even such a negative reading of the Catacombs indicates how powerful the skeletal contents could be to the visiting public. Whether or not one agreed with it, the sum was greater than its parts underground, where "these heaped-up bones, these tremendous clouds of nothingness!" could also serve as valuable human patrimony.[84]

Visitors to the Catacombs often identified with the space by casting forward in time and imagining themselves as future residents. For example, "three young people, who are between them forty-four years old," visited the Catacombs in 1810 because they wanted "to see what they will one day become."[85] Another guest surmised in July 1812 that "perhaps one day I will reside in this empire of death."[86] More humorously, F. De Oprey explained that "when one buys a house, they begin by visiting that house; this is what I did today; but this one won't cost me a thing."[87] Similarly, Fabien Pillet published a short poem in which he referred to the space as the "somber manor house" in which everyone would eventually sleep.[88] One of the more frequent refrains in the guestbook was for guests to bid a temporary farewell to the Catacombs, with the understanding that they would return after death. "I hope to return here," one visitor wrote in March 1811, "because there is nothing quite so sad as dying away from one's country."[89] Others were less sanguine, writing comments such as: "I won't be coming back to this somber place until someone carries me down." Or less realistically, "I hope that I won't come back here for two hundred years."[90] One could interpret these statements as run-of-the-mill memento mori, in which returning to the Catacombs is a euphemism for death more generally, but such pointed references to place seems to indicate how quickly the Catacombs had becoming an integral part of the city. Moreover, as placards throughout the tunnels reminded guests, the Catacombs was a continuously evolving and growing space: new bones had been transferred underground in 1804, 1809, 1811, 1813, and 1814. Indeed, it is quite possible that some of these early Catacombs visitors did eventually end up underground, since major Parisian cemeteries, including Père Lachaise, continued to supply the ossuary with new bones well into the twentieth century.[91]

Few of the French people who visited the Catacombs in the early nineteenth century were explicitly concerned with historical narratives, and they rarely expressed interest in formal political issues like the events and effects of the Revolution despite Héricart de Thury's hope that the ossuary would become an expiatory space. However, people were using the Catacombs to process and resolve some of the most difficult problems of the postrevolutionary era. Most notably they were working to belie the historical rupture of 1789 by envisioning an unbroken chain that connected the past, present, and future. For these people the Catacombs acted as a temporal link where one could "see people who are no more" and visit one's "future patrie."[92] When millions of Parisian bones embodied the French past, it was far from hostile. On the contrary, the subterranean population in the "Empire of Death" ultimately proved to be an unlikely source of communal identity and cohesion for the population living after the Terror.

Although Héricart de Thury's prediction that the "events of the Revolution" would draw crowds of mourners underground proved false, he was correct in assuming that the new Catacombs would provide a valuable space of contemplation for a population recovering from revolutionary dislocation. However, the ways in which visitors understood their descent underground varied greatly. For every individual who took advantage of a Catacombs tour to reflect on urgent political, social, or cultural concerns, there was someone in the wings stifling laughter. This chapter has offered a glimpse at the myriad, overlapping, and sometimes contrasting ways that Parisians used their Catacombs to confront and process some of the most difficult legacies of the Revolutionary era.

Spaces for the dead have a long history of bringing Parisians together. In the midst of the Wars of Religion, the Cemetery of the Innocents fostered a strong sense of civic identity based on a common religion and shared history.[93] During the equally tumultuous 1790s, citizens rallied around dead heroes, fallen martyrs and slain villains to assert a coherent republican identity. By the beginning of the nineteenth century, the Paris Catacombs stimulated a different sense of community that accommodated multiple ideological and religious perspectives. In this way, the Catacombs provided a comparably neutral alternative to more politicized spaces of memorialization. Vast new cemeteries like Père Lachaise effectively and beautifully housed the Parisian dead after 1804, but their overwhelming aesthetic was one of individuality and social stratification: the poor lay in plain common graves, the very wealthy purchased elaborately ornamented permanent tombs, while those in between enjoyed temporary five-year concessions. In elaborate public monuments like the Panthéon or the Mars Temple the state commemorated exceptional Frenchmen as national heroes and encouraged the revolutionary population to rally around them, but recent historians have argued that such "public pantheons" never effectively engaged the population in cohesive national sentiments because they ultimately amounted to little more than self-aggrandizing tools for insecure authorities.[94] By contrast, the masses of indistinguishable anonymous bones in the Catacombs offered a much more accurate and effective monument of the postrevolutionary capital: rich and poor, republican and royalist, past and present.

THE MUSEUM OF THE DEAD

From 1793 until 1816 a sculpture museum stood on Paris's left bank, across the river from the Louvre, in a former convent of Petits-Augustins nuns. Visitors to this museum, which by the summer of 1795 was known as the Museum of French Monuments, began their tour by entering an introductory hall that acclimated them to the museum's unique style and structure. This chamber was filled from floor to ceiling with historical sculptures and architectural fragments that the museum's director, Alexandre Lenoir, had collected from throughout the country. It featured works from the different epochs of France's long history, from pieces of ancient temples, to Cardinal Mazarin's (empty) mausoleum. Guests next passed into a room displaying funerary monuments that once belonged the oldest French monarchs—Childebert, Pepin the Short, and Hugues Capet. Once they finished examining these historically remote artifacts, an elaborately decorated fourteenth-century "gothic" room awaited, with the looming (empty) mausoleum of Charles V and Jeanne de Bourbon as its centerpiece. Fifteenth-, sixteenth-, and seventeenth-century rooms followed suit, until guests were finally directed toward an exterior court-yard, the "Elysian Garden," where the entombed remains of Molière, Descartes, Abélard, and Héloïse sat, surrounded by more tombs, sarcoph-agi, trees, and assorted greenery. The overall effect of the museum and its garden was supposed to be one of total historical immersion and educa-tion. When crossing the threshold to the Museum of French Monuments, visitors stepped out of Paris's eleventh arrondissement and into its past.

Clearly, this was more than a museum dedicated to history and sculp-ture; it was also a vast and unprecedented display of the Old Regime's material culture of death. As one visitor described it at the beginning of the nineteenth century, the Museum of French Monuments had effectively embraced and re-created "the sepulchral history of France."[1] At every turn, visitors encountered traces of the dead, whose tombs, effigies, and mausolea occupied the most prominent places throughout the museum. Although each room contained a range of monuments, it was these sundry burial chambers that caught visitors' eyes and engaged their imaginations. Sometimes this was due to the sheer size of the monuments: Cardinal Richelieu's mausoleum was fourteen feet long and stood six feet tall in the seventeenth-century room. In other instances specific tombs set the tone and style for the rest of the room, such as the fifteenth-century room, in which "the ceiling, the casements of the windows, and all the decorative parts of the apartment [were] shaped after the model of the tomb of Louis XII," which stood at its center.[2] The overall effect of so many spaces filled with—and defined by—tombs could be morose, but as the British poet (and supporter of the Revolution) Helen Maria Williams noted, such a gloomy tone suited the feelings she felt when contemplating "the mortal-ity of ages" and corresponded with the "sentiments of awe and venera-tion" with which she viewed "the relics of the illustrious dead."[3]

Despite the ubiquity of death in the museum, scholars have gener-ally overlooked this macabre feature, opting instead to focus on Lenoir's prominent, but contentious, place in the history of museums and histori-cal representation.[4] In the only monograph to focus exclusively on the museum, Alexandra Stara discusses the historical significance of having real artifacts on display, and while she distinguishes between "commemo-rative" and "non-commemorative" pieces in the museum, she neglects to unpack the significance that so many of these commemorative sculptures were in fact tombs that had been emptied of their corporeal contents.[5]

This chapter resolves this discrepancy and focuses on the key role that the dead played in this strange museum where they were simultaneously present and absent. The actual remains of the dead were for the most part missing from the museum—many of them lay tangled and decomposing in a mass grave behind Saint-Denis cathedral, about thirteen kilometers north of the museum. However, this absence was central to the museum's identity as a space of history. Entombed kings had been the literal embodiment of hereditary power under the Old Regime, but once they were emptied of their sacred contents and relocated to an institutional setting, these same tombs became artifacts that provided visitors with access to a thousand years of French history.

The Museum of French Monuments may seem like an odd companion to sites like Père Lachaise Cemetery and the Paris Catacombs. It was short lived, low on actual corpses, and featured the exceptional instead of the ordinary dead, but this chapter argues that it functioned in a similar way to these more prominent spaces. Specifically, the museum challenged old hierarchies and provided new opportunities for social cohesion. By cataloguing, describing, and displaying discarded tombs from France's pre-revolutionary years, Alexandre Lenoir offered visitors to his museum an alternative narrative of their nation's past, which reconciled the rupture of revolution with a need for history. The generations of tombs on display throughout the museum provided material evidence of a common history while the emptiness of those tombs reminded visitors at every turn of the Revolution's violent rejection of that past. Meanwhile, the savants who occupied the tombs in the Elysian Garden exemplified individual genius as well as the enduring art of fraternal and romantic love. In both their conspicuous absence inside the museum and their unexpected presence in its backyard, the dead were at the heart of the museum's appeal and effectiveness as a (post)revolutionary space.

The museum also shared the Catacombs' and cemeteries' heterotopian ability to confuse boundaries of space, time, and social rank. At its most elemental, the museum was an accumulation of fragments displaced from churches throughout the country. The dozens of tombs were most obviously out of place, having spent decades, in some cases, centuries, concealed from public view in subterranean crypts. For the museum's critics, this displacement stripped these objects of their context and robbed them of authenticity and meaning. By contrast, Lenoir argued that the act of reassembling and displaying thousands of disparate pieces, gave them a powerful new meaning as components in a great national story, in effect providing them with a new, more socially responsible context. By resituating them in a space that was open to the public two days a week, Lenoir made the exceptional and previously sacred dead, quite literally, accessible. As Louis-Sébastien Mercier described it in 1797: "I walked on tombs, I strode over mausoleums. Every rank, every costume, every crown was beneath my feet. . . . Lowered from their pedestals the grandest personages were brought down to my level; I could touch their brows, their mouths, speak in Richelieu's ear, and interrogate Turenne and Mallebranche."[6] For all of its violence and destruction, the Revolution had made possible this grand and equalizing spectacle. Like Père Lachaise Cemetery and the Paris Catacombs, the Museum of French Monuments used the dead to create a new kind of space in the city—a microworld that contained centuries, made sense of an otherwise problematic past, and provided a consoling image of the future.

Rescuing the Past

The Museum of French Monuments began as the solution to a revolutionary conundrum. It was the product of dual revolutionary impulses to destroy the Old Regime while preserving its cultural patrimony. After the National Assembly nationalized church property and dissolved monastic orders in the first year of the Revolution, it recognized a need to protect the many historic and artistic treasures contained on these properties, particularly those that they deemed "worthy of embellishing the territory of a free people."[7] To this end, the Committee of Public Instruction created the Commission of Monuments in 1790 to seek out objects of this nature throughout Paris. They also established a series of temporary depots in the city to house valuable works of art, sculpture, music, literature, and mechanical science. An October 1790 decree founded the largest of these depots—primarily for pieces of sculpture—in the former convent of the Petits-Augustins nuns.

From its earliest incarnation the Petits-Augustins depot was under the direction of an ambitious young artist named Alexandre Lenoir. Like so many individuals who made their names during this time, Lenoir was by all accounts an unremarkable figure until the Revolution opened up new opportunities for him. He was born to a family of merchants in Paris on December 27, 1761, and received a standard bourgeois education at the Collège Mazarin. After graduating, Lenoir decided to pursue a career as an artist and enrolled in the Royal Academy in 1778 to study under one of the king's painters, Gabriel-François Doyen. Lenoir's relationship with Doyen was the fortuitous connection that placed him in a position of power once the Revolution began, as Doyen was a member of the Commission of Monuments and pushed to have his pupil involved in the group's work. When the commission was looking to hire a permanent guardian in June 1791 for the Petits-Augustins depot, Doyen used his personal relationship with the mayor of Paris (Sylvain Bailly) to land Lenoir this prestigious position. Although the appointment of such an inexperienced administrator raised heckles among members of the commission, Lenoir immediately threw himself into his new job. During his first six months, Lenoir went through hundreds of items from the monasteries of Paris, such as mausoleums, statues, epitaphs, and tableaus.[8] He then collected and catalogued more and more material as it became the property of the revolutionary state, including content from former churches, the homes of wealthy émigrés, and other notable properties such as the Sorbonne. When municipal administrators showed up to Petits-Augustins in July 1791 they were amazed by the work that Lenoir had carried out so quickly and efficiently, noting that the contents of his depot were "perfectly in order, ticketed, and numbered."[9]

Lenoir was a meticulous revolutionary administrator, but he shied away from the tumultuous politics of his time. His interest in maintaining his position at the depot took precedence over any ideology that he may have privately held.[10] Professionally and publicly, he behaved as many French citizens of his era probably did: he pledged allegiance to the prevailing political order, whatever that happened to be. He began his career as a moderate republican artist, cooperated with the Jacobin government, but denounced radicalism during the Directory. After 1799 he eagerly supported Bonaparte but quickly switched his allegiance to the returning Bourbons in 1815 and lived out the rest of his life as a distinguished Chevalier in the Legion of Honor. In contrast to his politics, however, Lenoir was remarkably consistent in his devotion to his museum's collection and to its tombs in particular. He internalized his professional duty to such a degree that his identity quickly became synonymous with the rescue, preservation, and protection of damaged art. In 1798, an acquaintance teased Lenoir about his attachment to the museum and its macabre contents, urging him to "come out from your lugubrious tombs, which, despite their extreme love and gratitude for your care cannot express their feelings like *bon vivants*."[11] Similarly, an English travel writer who made Lenoir's acquaintance early in the nineteenth century described how, when in Lenoir's company, "I fancy the illustrious dead are present in all their majesty around him. Grave, silent, and pensive, his character and manner strongly impress you with the idea of an affectionate son, who collects with tender care, the ashes of his murdered parent."[12] When the restored Bourbon monarchy finally closed down the museum in 1816, Lenoir followed these "parents" back to Saint-Denis, where he became the head administrator in charge of their restoration.

But back in 1793, a young Lenoir was just getting started. Although he'd been guardian of Petits-Augustins for two years, the laws and practices of the Terror brought new urgency to this role. Most radically, the National Assembly issued a decree in October 1793 that ordered the destruction of all emblems of feudalism, including statues, signs, and other symbols of the past. This coupled with the radical campaign of de-Christianization led to the widespread destruction of churches and vacant estates throughout the country and prompted the Abbé Grégoire to coin the neologism "vandalism" a year later.[13] While some of this destruction had practical and economic motivations—anything made out of lead could be reconfigured into bullets, for example—such violence against the decorative vestiges of the past was a deeply symbolic act. Lenoir found himself in an awkward position during the Terror: As a revolutionary administrator, he needed to profess his hatred of the Old Regime, yet as someone working for the preservation of monuments, he also wanted to protect the artistic products of that regime. Lenoir found himself acting out this tension in person as he defended various monuments from what he later called "the axe of the Vandals" (figure 5.1).[14] The most famous early example of this occurred in December 1793, when angry sans-culottes invaded the Sorbonne and attacked the mausoleum of Cardinal Richelieu, which had been carved by the celebrated seventeenth-century sculptor François Girardon. Lenoir placed his body between the mausoleum and the angry crowd, whom he subsequently described as

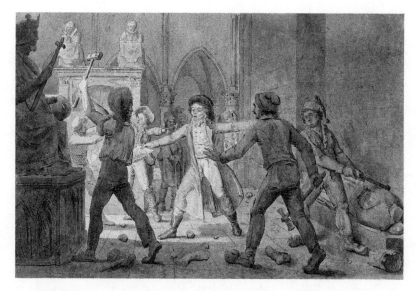

Figure 5.1. "Alexandre Lenoir Defending the Monuments of the Abbey of Saint-Denis." Musée du Louvre, RMN-Grand Palais/Art Resource NY.

"enemies of the arts" and perpetrators of "barbarianism, ignorance, and cruelty."[15] Lenoir was famously injured during this standoff—he suffered a stab wound from a bayonet to his hand—but he successfully protected the mausoleum from total destruction. Richelieu's mummified corpse on the other hand was decapitated and paraded before an angry crowd.[16]

The dramatic rescue operation of the Richelieu tomb illustrates Lenoir's early mandate to preserve valuable works of art, but it also demonstrates the vast difference between the dead and the monuments that contained them. Obliterating the physical remains of men like Richelieu—who exemplified prerevolutionary power—while saving their tombs helped revolutionaries resolve the tension implicit in their mission to both destroy and preserve the past. It allowed them to stake out a radical position against certain elements of the Old Regime (absolutism) while preserving others (artistic genius). The illustrious dead made especially good targets for destruction because of their symbolic weight as the actual embodiment of hereditary privilege and royal authority.[17] This same phenomenon played out in a more extreme form in the summer and fall of 1793 when dozens of kings, queens, and other notables were exhumed from the

Saint-Denis Abbey, just north of Paris. Lenoir was present for both phases of this disinterment, with a mandate to preserve anything of artistic or historic value. The significance of the task was certainly not lost on Lenoir, who enjoyed the "most extraordinary experience" of watching all of the "disfigured" and decomposing kings pass before his eyes, an experience he blithely described as "piquant."[18] At the end of this lengthy process, Lenoir had secured dozens of tombs for his depot, from the seventh to the eighteenth centuries. The remains of the royal families and other dignitaries were all thrown together in mass graves behind the abbey and covered in quicklime to hasten their decomposition.

The royal tombs raised the profile of the Petits-Augustins depot, but their presence also made it more controversial, particularly in the politically charged climate of 1793–94. Lenoir needed to position himself as someone who could protect the tombs as artifacts without revering them as repositories of sacred kingship. For example, in his report of the exhumation, he described the surreal experience of watching a perfectly mummified Henri IV emerge from his tomb: "I took his hands with a certain respect, which I do not have to defend because I am a true republican."[19] The Committee of Public Instruction saw the value of Lenoir's collection and even requested that he open the depot to the public from August 10 to September 30, 1793, in honor of the first anniversary of the republic. Yet, when Lenoir petitioned the committee a year later to have this museumlike status renewed and made permanent, they demurred on the grounds that Petits-Augustins contained too many images of "tyrants and their families" and religious items designed to lie and confuse the people of France.[20] In short, the past was still too dangerous to the fledgling republic.

Contrary to this concern, many of the earliest visitors to the Petits-Augustins depot interpreted the space as a sublime representation of the Revolution, not the Old Regime. Most famously, Louis-Sébastien Mercier reveled in the museum as "the veritable mirror of our revolution" with all of its "contrasts . . . bizarre rapprochements . . . [and] singular chaos!" Using language that presaged future conversations about the Catacombs, Mercier celebrated the fact that ancient "pagan" statues stood next to Christian ones in the depot, and that a bust of the seventeenth-century playwright Racine leaned for support against the tomb of sixth-century Merovingian queen Frédégonde. He delighted in the "confusion of centuries" that collapsed history and offered unprecedented opportunities for "contemplative spectators" to reflect on big concepts like mortality, power, and inequality.[21] On the opposite end of the political spectrum, René de Chateaubriand made a similar observation, while coming to a very different conclusion. In the first volume of *Mémoires d'outre-tomb* Chateaubriand used Petits-Augustins and its "collection of ruins and tombs from all centuries, thrown together pêle-mêle" as a metaphor for a more general sense of social disorder and degeneration after the Revolution.[22] For better or for worse, the sepulchral contents of the Petits-Augustins depot intimately tied it to the tumult of the Revolution.

Completing the Collection

As the Terror came to a close and Thermidorian republicans searched for new ways to carry out their instructional mission, they began directing more support and resources toward Lenoir's depot. In October 1795 the Committee of Public Instruction passed a law that officially redesignated Petits-Augustins as the Museum of French Monuments. With a new name came new responsibilities: instead of providing temporary refuge to valuable pieces of sculpture, Petits-Augustins now needed to be useful to the population of Paris and France. Lenoir quickly developed a dual mandate for the museum: it would educate the people of France about the two subjects contained within its walls: art and history. Once his project officially shifted from taking up transitory to permanent space, Lenoir also reconfigured his own role as the museum's director. Instead of simply salvaging, preserving, and cataloguing, Lenoir took it upon himself to reconceptualize the contents of Petits-Augustins as a "collection" that presented a coherent story of the nation's past, and thereby fulfilled an important function for a population reeling from the destruction and dislocation of the Terror. His museum would do the important work of fostering collective identity by putting the nation's history on display. As he explained in the preface to a 1795 description of the museum, a visit to this space would inspire French citizens with hatred for tyranny, respect for the law, sorrow for the difficulties that France faced and above all, love for the patrie. He imagined how his guests would cry out, overwhelmed by enthusiasm: "How happy I am to have been born French."[23]

Alongside this new purpose for his museum, Lenoir's stated motivation for acquiring content changed. He was no longer satisfied to merely rescue and preserve endangered pieces of art in the capital; now he needed to grow his collection in order to "complete" it. This quickly expanded Lenoir's reach well beyond Paris as he sought out historically significant monuments—often tombs—that had been scattered during the Terror. For example, in 1796 Lenoir heard about the imperiled tomb of Diane de Poitiers—a prominent sixteenth-century courtier and mistress to Henry II. The tomb was located about a hundred kilometers southwest of Paris, in Eure-et-Loire, on the property of a drink seller named Antoine Saliar. Saliar had purchased the tomb at auction in 1794 and was known to be using it as a trough to feed his animals when it came to Lenoir's attention two years later. The tomb was particularly appealing to Lenoir because it would complete a triptych for his sixteenth-century room. "Citizen minister," Lenoir wrote to the minister of the interior in June, "if you permit me this monument, I will reunite in my museum, the tombs of the lover, the mistress, and their daughter." Saliar was willing to part with the sarcophagi for three hundred francs, and Lenoir quickly arranged for its transfer to Paris.[24] Lenoir's archives are filled with these types of acquisitions and exchanges, whereby he attempted to rectify the Revolution's hasty divestment of church contents to private individuals and bring them back into the public domain.[25]

Lenoir's zeal for building up his collection sometimes led to tense interactions with regional administrators whose interests were at odds with his own. In the year X (1801–2) Lenoir attempted to acquire the sixteenth-century tombs of Henri de Guise and his spouse, Catherine of Clèves, which were located in a church in the northern seaside commune of Eu. In his initial request to the minister of the interior, Lenoir justified this acquisition as a rescue mission: he claimed that the tombs were in danger because of their proximity to a market, which exposed them to many indifferent and clumsy passersby. What if a market goer spilled something on the tombs and knocked them over? he asked the minister, Jérome-Antoine Chaptal. Chaptal initially agreed, but once the departmental prefect, Jacques-Claude Beugnot, heard about the monument's impending "rescue," he quickly sent letters of protest to both Lenoir and Chaptal. In his letter to Lenoir, Beugnot explained that the tombs were his department's only historical monument and one that they wished to keep. He further noted that if Lenoir were to transport the tombs to Paris, he would undoubtedly have to break the monument into pieces, thereby continuing the "impious work of the barbarians" who, during the Revolution, had stripped the monument of its precious metals.[26] When communicating directly with the minister of the interior, Beugnot was much more critical of Lenoir's project. He acknowledged Lenoir's fine work in rescuing endangered pieces of art during the Revolution but reminded Chaptal that the tombs in question were in excellent condition; they had even been recently repaired by the local government. These were hardly the displaced, abandoned, and isolated monuments that Lenoir described. He further explained that the church in question had been built specifically for the preservation of the two tombs it contained. To move these tombs to Paris, he explained, would strip them of meaning, since a sterile museum environment could never duplicate the traditions, memories, and history of a community's devotion.[27]

For Lenoir, the local significance of a tomb was always secondary to the role it could play in his museum. By removing them from their original contexts, Lenoir promised to give these monuments a new and more important role to play. He explained that the Guise tombs would have had a natural resting place with the sixteenth-century Valois tombs already contained in the museum. In his complaint to Chaptal, Beugnot referred to this intention, noting that the tombs were of little aesthetic value to the museum, which already featured an abundance of sixteenth-century monuments. He astutely countered, "I may be mistaken, but isn't it the history of art, and not the history of France that [Lenoir] wishes to write?"[28] Lenoir ultimately lost the fight: Chaptal instructed him to stay away from Eu and reminded him that the museum's mandate did not extend beyond endangered pieces, and certainly excluded monuments that communes wished to keep. By rebuking Lenoir in this way both the prefect and Chaptal highlighted the main transformation that had taken place in Lenoir's understanding of the museum since 1793. As he acquired more monuments and came closer to "completing" his collection, Lenoir became increasingly interested in using his museum to evoke the past and to present a coherent historical narrative to his visitors.

Lenoir's ambition to complete his collection has made his work controversial since the end of the eighteenth century. Twentieth-century scholars dubbed him a fanatic, a thief, and even a vandal.[29] He also earned a bad reputation among several of his contemporaries, including the famous artist

and critic responsible for the restoration of the Panthéon during the Revolution, Antoine Quatremère de Quincy, who attacked Lenoir for continuing to amass monuments in his museum long after emergency conservation
was necessary. In a scathing critique published in year VIII (1800), Quatremère de Quincy accused Lenoir of directing a "cemetery for the arts"
in his "so-called conservatory."[30] In a similarly themed invective, written in 1806 but not published until the Restoration he urged Lenoir to
"stop pretending that artworks are preserved in those depositories. You
may have carried the material hull there," he spat, "but it is doubtful you
transferred the network of ideas and relations that made the works alive
with interest." Invoking Lenoir's collection of funerary sculpture in particular, he concluded, "What do those effigies which are now mere matter
mean to me? What are those mausolea without a proper resting place,
those cenotaphs twice empty, these graves that even death has deserted?"[31]
In *Genius of Christianity*, Chateaubriand similarly chastised the museum
for "destroying" the "ancient sepulchers of France" by tearing them out of
context and making them "subservient only to the history of the arts."[32]

To critics like Quatremère de Quincy and Chateaubriand, the act of
removing a tomb from its original setting when it was not actually in
danger was an act of violence that robbed the particular monument of
its significance or meaning. Of course, Lenoir completely disagreed with
this assessment because he understood his project as a conscious act of
construction, not just conservation. This also explains why he regularly
created his own monuments for the museum, items he called "fabriques,"
by combining debris from several unrelated statues. For example, Lenoir
crafted a tomb for Charles V and his wife, Jeanne de Bourbon out of "debris from several monuments" from the fourteenth century that he had
proudly "brought together."[33] Similarly, when Lenoir was missing a bust
or statue of an individual who he thought was particularly historically
relevant, he simply commissioned his friends and colleagues to "create"
a new monument out of scrap pieces of marble that he had on hand.
Quatremère de Quincy was predictably outraged by this kind of work and
accused Lenoir of creating "mutilated art."[34] However, for Lenoir, it was
necessary to complete individual pieces in his museum in order to create a
coherent whole, regardless of so-called authenticity.[35]

These were not Alexandre Lenoir's only critics; for others, he was a
shameless packrat, incapable of distinguishing masterpieces from dreck.

In 1802 the editors of the *Journal des Arts, des sciences, et de littérature* published an anonymous letter in which the author attacked the museum as a useless waste of state resources. The author, "an impartial art lover," centered his critique on two related points: first, the museum had outlived its purpose as a temporary depot and second, that its indiscriminate conservation of bad and mediocre art alongside works of genius was counterproductive. According to the author, Petits-Augustins had been tolerable as a temporary depot, but as a museum it was badly in need of an aesthete's hand to weed out the mediocre and the bad, since "the goal of such an establishment is to instruct young devotees of the Arts, to shape their good taste, and to offer up the very best models" for emulation. In particular, the author opposed the stodgy tombs and statues that dated from the Gothic period, which he considered the nadir of French art. Such objects, "of no artistic value" belonged in a churchyard somewhere, where naïve visitors would not mistake them for art. The editors of the *Journal des Arts* published this scathing critique so that they could refute it, point by point. They chastised the author for his short-sighted and outdated attitudes and for his narrow understanding of Lenoir's project. "Always with the young Artists and young Sculptors!" they mocked, "perhaps the author might consider a different kind of sculptor, one whose works last much longer than marble: *historians.*" They explained how historians would visit the museum's tombs in order to study the crimes and virtues of the dead. Unlike art students, these scholars could see past the fancy exteriors of elaborate stonework to recognize the truth of the past, however unpleasant. "The Augustins Museum is useful," they concluded, "because it conserves for history, for contemporaries, and for posterity" objects that would otherwise be lost forever.[36] By invoking history, the journal editors clarified what had quickly become one of the museum's main priorities. By the end of the century, Lenoir had moved far beyond preservation; by then he was energetically working to use his museum to (re)construct the past.

"The Sepulchral History of France"

When Lenoir spoke about completing his museum's collection, he usually referenced his need to acquire pieces from all eras in French history. For example, in 1795 when he requested permission to retrieve a handful of monuments that remained in the Saint-Denis abbey, including four tombs belonging to ("Saint") Louis IX's immediate family, Lenoir noted that these pieces were particularly valuable to him because his museum was lacking in thirteenth-century content.[37] His collection needed to be comprehensive because one of his goals from the museum's earliest days was to "represent the history of the nation through the monuments themselves."[38] To this end, Lenoir worked throughout the latter half of the 1790s to convert his once-provisional depot into a totally immersive experience that would envelope visitors in the past and guide them through their nation's history. Meanwhile, Lenoir continually wrote and published catalogues, descriptions, and essays that described and analyzed the museum's contents, most notably an eight-volume illustrated description, published between 1800 and 1806.[39] These documents brought the museum to those who couldn't visit Paris, but they also provided a narrative framework for an otherwise unwieldy collection.[40] Reading these descriptions alongside contemporary reflections on the museum from those who toured it provides valuable insight into the historical narrative that Lenoir hoped to craft with his project as well as the meaning that visitors intuited from the space, regardless of its founder's intention.

Lenoir was adamant about the Museum of French Monuments' pedagogical value. As he explained in 1800, he sought to present the collection from two perspectives: the political and the pedagogical. "From the political perspective," he wrote, "[the museum] must be established with enough splendor and magnificence to speak to all eyes, and draw curious parties from all four corners of the earth." While "from the perspective of public instruction, it must contain all that the arts and sciences together might offer to public education."[41] Lenoir had always been interested in using the museum to represent the history of art in France, but he was equally preoccupied with using art to piece together a more general history of the nation. To meet this objective, Lenoir decided very early on to organize his collection chronologically, with a room dedicated to each epoch in French history. The original October 1795 decree from the Committee of Public Instruction that granted museum status on the Petits-Augustins depot even specified that the monuments on display would be organized chronologically.[42] By this "reasoned and thoughtful" arrangement, Lenoir asserted, the museum would be at once beautiful, interesting and didactic.[43] One of the museum's earliest champions, Louis-Sébastien

Mercier lamented this shift toward order and decried the loss of the depot's "poetic disorder" in favor of an "insipid and monotonous regularity" that left him cold.[44] However, for Lenoir, a chronological mode of
organization seemed logical and natural. "If one considers the chronology
of past centuries like an open textbook in which the sequence of events
can be read," he wrote "one senses the necessity of classifying the monuments according to their epochs, following the borders that nature herself
drew."[45]

The chronological organization of the museum was so important to
Lenoir that he fought to maintain strict personal control over it. His intense personal investment was on full display in the winter of 1801–2,
when he clashed with the museum's recently appointed architect, Pierre
Moreau. The affair began when Moreau wrote to Minister of the Interior
Chaptal to explain that a slight "difficulty" had arisen between himself
and Lenoir. Although the whole purpose of the museum having a devoted architect was for Lenoir to share his workload, Moreau soon found
Lenoir to be extremely controlling of every aspect of the museum's management and operation, only allowing the architect to work on large construction projects. To address the problem, Chaptal drafted a polite letter
to Lenoir and reminded him that certain demarcation lines needed to exist
in the museum in order for it to function efficiently. He explained that
ideally, Lenoir would direct the restoration of statues, mausoleums, and
mutilated pieces of sculpture, but that Moreau would oversee the placement of pieces throughout the museum and set the overall tone of each
room. Lenoir shot back a reply unequivocally repudiating this "gravely
unjust" division of labor. He reminded the minister that without his constant work and research, the museum would be entirely without character
or truth. "I am the creator of this unique establishment," Lenoir boldly
asserted, "it is the object of all of my cares and concerns. To rob me of the
pleasure of organizing my 'centuries' according to the styles of their age is
to completely destroy the appeal of my work."[46] Moreau left the museum
several months later.

In addition to a chronological retelling of French history, Lenoir built
his museum to convey a specific narrative about the history of French
art. He carefully planned each room to demonstrate a clear artistic and
architectural style, often exaggerating stylistic differences so that visitors
would be able to easily observe the "immense gaps" that existed from one

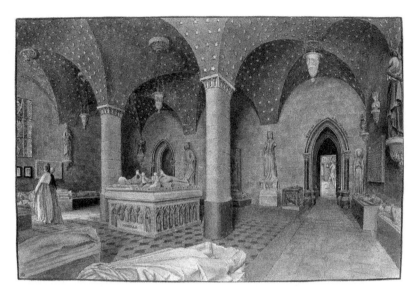

Figure 5.2. Alexandre Lenoir, "Thirteenth-century Room in the Museum of French Monuments." Musée du Louvre, RMN-Grand Palais/Art Resource NY.

century to another.[47] But he intended his visitors to experience more than just art historical trends. For example, when guests entered the room dedicated to the early middle ages, Lenoir wanted to overwhelm them with feelings of oppression and obscurity. He used the debris from Saint-Denis to build a heavy, dimly lit room with a low vaulted ceiling painted dark blue and speckled with stars (see figure 5.2). When the famous German writer Auguste von Kotzebue visited the Museum of French Monuments for the first time in 1804 he described how "an oppressive sensation seized me upon stepping into that closet" with its "kings and queens, hewn out of rude masses of stones, with folded hands."[48] Lenoir intended this room to convey a sense of weakness that resulted from the magic and superstition of the domineering medieval church.[49] As guests progressed through the museum, passing from century to century, they would experience more light and more refined works of art. When they reached the sixteenth-century room, they found it bathed in light and color, featuring ninety-five monuments, including high-quality tombs with realistic sculptures of the dead monarchs. Lenoir was especially proud of the restored tombs of Henri II and his spouse Catherine de Medici, which he believed were crafted with such skill that onlookers would unavoidably be moved by profound sensibility.[50] Visitors to the museum were similarly impressed by the tomb of Francis I and queen Claudia, which featured marble sculptures of royal couple, "longer than their natural size, extended as corpses" in which the artist (Jean Goujon) "finely expressed the privation of life in the countenance and muscles."[51]

A number of art historians have noted the overtly political agenda driving this organization. In general, Lenoir's interpretation of the history of art in France directly contradicted the prerevolutionary consensus, which charted a gradual improvement of art until Louis XIV in the seventeenth century, when it became perpetually sustained through the French Academy. In the museum, Lenoir adjusted this timeline so that the sixteenth-century French Renaissance became the high point, to be followed by two hundred years of degradation under Bourbon rule.[52] Describing the era of Francis I in one of his catalogues, Lenoir explained that by studying the monuments from this period visitors to his museum would come to the obvious conclusion that the Renaissance had clearly been the pinnacle of French artistic achievement.[53] While Louis XIV had tried very hard a century later to re-create the accomplishments of the Renaissance through the royal academies, Lenoir explained that encouragement alone could not make artists. In order to thrive, he wrote, art required unblemished public morals, good government, and artistic freedom. In Lenoir's history, Louis XIV's artists were little more than decadent sycophants; one glance at the museum's seventeenth-century room would reveal the uniformity and lack of originality in art during this time. He remained convinced that after examining the museum's "methodologically classified" monuments, it would be virtually impossible to dispute that the arts declined in France after the Bourbon ascendancy.[54]

Fans of the museum appreciated Lenoir's work on art history, but they also expressed interest in a more straightforward history of their nation. After the publication of the first installment of his descriptive account of the museum in 1800, supporters of Lenoir's work requested that he include a chronology of French kings in his second volume. He obliged and volume 2 opened with a ninety-eight-page introductory essay on the genealogy of French kings, complete with engravings of their likeness on coins.[55] However, Lenoir "augmented" this essay with a copy of his twenty-six-page eyewitness testimony describing the exhumations that had taken place at the Saint-Denis Abbey in the fall of 1793. Within the span of a hundred pages, readers could learn, for example, that Francis I was the "restorer of arts and letters in France," the father of seven children, and in a state of "liquid putrefaction" by the time his tomb was opened in 1793.[56]

The intention behind Lenoir's published description of the exhumations is difficult to pin down. It is a stark and dispassionate account of how dozens of elite and royal bodies were removed from their tombs over the course of two weeks, from October 12 to 25, 1793. There was a vaguely educational and "scientific" tone to this document, which superficially evaluated various methods of mummification and stages of decomposition. For example, it described General Turenne (d. 1675) and Henri IV (d. 1610) as perfectly preserved but noted how most of the corpses from the mid-seventeenth to the mid-eighteenth century were so badly decayed and oozing with stinking black liquid, that they made the workers who disinterred them sick with fever and diarrhea.[57] Lenoir also sketched the dead kings during their exhumation; he never published these grisly images but did show them to friends and interested visitors (see figure 5.3). This catalogue of royal decomposition seems like a powerful act of desacralization. In the wake of a revolution that tore down centuries of monarchic rule, it is difficult not to read more into Lenoir's statement that Hugues Capet's father (d. 956) had been "almost reduced to dust."[58] What could be a better symbol of an obsolete monarchy than its actual physical degradation?

The Saint-Denis exhumations also point to another key feature of the museum: that its own origin story was just as powerful as the national narrative it presented to readers and audiences. Lenoir never shied away from his museum's controversial beginnings. The first sentences of the 1810 installment of his book series about the museum noted that "the destruction of artistic monuments is the necessary consequence of political disorders."[59] In the stormy excitement of a revolutionary environment, he explained, people were easily carried away with a desire to avenge past wrongs, but it was the duty of a wise government to implement safeguards—like Petits-Augustins—to protect public monuments. While his audience mostly appreciated the museum's conservationist work, they

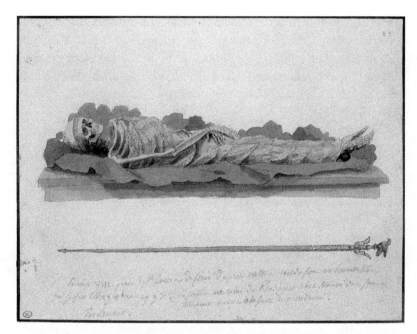

Figure 5.3. Alexandre Lenoir, "The Remains of Louis VIII, Exhumed from His Tomb in 1793." Musée du Louvre, RMN-Grand Palais/Art Resource NY.

couldn't help but reflect on the violence that made it necessary. Most visitors to the Museum of French Monuments knew that the historic tombs that filled its rooms were empty and they knew why. As Louis-Sébastien Mercier described it in 1797, "after years of repose, the kings felt the blows of this incredible revolution."[60] Even authors of otherwise glowing descriptions of the museum punctuated their narratives with references to the museum's controversial origins. Helen Maria Williams referred to "jacobinical fury" and made special notes about which tombs and monuments had "had suffered most from the reign of terror."[61] Anne Plumptre similarly expounded on the "phrensy of destruction" that had gripped France in 1793, "to be communicated from one person to another, from one province to another, with the rapidity of a contagion."[62] Many others, including Kotzebue and Yorke, included in their descriptions of the museum vivid details about the Saint-Denis exhumations, paraphrased directly from Lenoir's eyewitness testimony. In this way, visitors—even those broadly sympathetic to Revolutionary goals—used the museum to access a difficult era. Not only did it provide a vivid narrative of art and history in France, it also offered an opportunity to revisit one of the most spectacular examples of revolutionary violence, one in which "those barbarous Iconoclasts" engaged in the state-sanctioned "arts of destruction."[63] The museum's chronology of France stopped at the seventeenth century, but the history and provenance of its content continually invoked the very recent and problematic past.

But reflecting on violence was not the same thing as repudiating the Revolution. Indeed, many of the visitors who shook their heads at the memory of the Terror also applauded the museum for facilitating reconciliation and reunion in its aftermath. Most obviously, the museum brought together under its roof a thousand years of history and made that history intelligible to a diverse postrevolutionary audience. One of France's most significant nineteenth-century historians, Jules Michelet, famously recalled how when he was a child his mother regularly brought him to the museum where he passed from room to room, excited and eagerly in pursuit of knowledge about bygone eras.[64] The British radical and writer Anne Plumptre reacted similarly: she appreciated the museum's fine order and its uncanny ability to unite "in the same space, and at the same moment in time" a diverse collection of people from across history. However, she took this theme a step further when marveling at the social difference evident among the museum's local visitors. Visiting the museum on days designated for the public, rather than by appointment, was an edifying enterprise, she explained, because "the rooms are then thronged by a motley concourse of all ranks and descriptions of persons, all preserving the most exact order, and presenting the extraordinary spectacle of the most ignorant and the most enlightened uniting in equal notes of admiration."[65] Not only did the museum bring together the past and present, the living and the dead, it struck some sympathetic visitors as a delightfully heterogeneous social space—a not-so-subtle reflection of revolutionary social reorganization.

Lenoir also took advantage of his museum's intimate rapport with the Revolution to explicitly foster reconciliation between the past and the present. For example, in the summer of 1803, he arranged an unusual nighttime tour of the museum for members of the Institut de France, including the celebrated author Jacques-Henri Bernardin de Saint-Pierre and his spouse. Handheld torches added a "solemn effect" to the tour that was further exaggerated by a group of musicians Lenoir had commissioned to play funeral dirges as guests entered each of the tomb filled chambers. One participant of the tour described how the music, "with the surrounding monuments, the numerous torches, and all the decorations of these sacred repositories filled my mind with indescribable sensations."[66] This type of commemorative event was exactly what the revolutionary government had feared when they refused Lenoir's 1793 request to transform Petits-Augustins from a provisional depot into a museum, but a decade later the political climate had changed quite significantly, as had the population's relationship with the Revolution and the Old Regime. By the beginning of the nineteenth century, the past (whether recent or distant) no longer posed an immediate threat to the present. Instead, as spaces like the Catacombs and the Museum of French Monuments illustrate, it was rapidly becoming a desirable and useful place to visit.

History's Backyard Cemetery

Lenoir removed kings from their "permanent" resting places, disposed of their remains, and hauled their empty tombs back to the Museum of French Monuments. In the museum, he organized the tombs, mausoleums, and pieces of reclaimed statues and sculpture to render France's monarchic past legible to a population reeling from revolution and historical rupture. However, there was one part of the museum that he excluded from this narrative. Once visitors to the Museum of French Monuments had passed through each of France's centuries, Lenoir invited them to step outside of the museum, outside of history, and into the museum's large garden, where he had established his own personal cemetery, which he called the Elysian Garden (see figure 5.4). Lenoir had been planning a burial garden for his museum since the summer of 1796, when he asked the minister of the interior for permission to construct a green space that would act as a "public promenade" for the museum's visitors.[67] Six months later he was already referring to this garden as an "elysée," but it was not until 1799 that Lenoir started to actively collect the bones, hearts, and ashes of France's illustrious dead. The garden was one of Lenoir's proudest achievements, it contained the remains of seven "illustrious figures," notable for their contributions to French philosophy and literature. Years

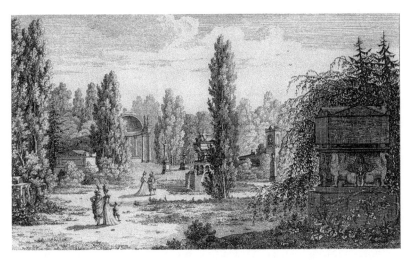

Figure 5.4. Alexandre Lenoir and Laurent Guyot, "View of the 'Elysée' Garden from 'Museum of French Monuments Volume 5.'" Musée du Louvre, RMN-Grand Palais/Art Resource NY.

after the museum closed, Lenoir recalled it fondly as "a garden whose varied and picturesque plantation lent it the character of an Elysium as conceived by a poetic imagination. . . . Everything in the Elysium spoke to the soul, excited daydreams and enthusiasm."[68]

Lenoir's concept for the garden reflected contemporary ideas about death, commemoration, and landscape architecture. Since the traditional cemetery had become unacceptable in France in the second half of the eighteenth century, reformers, artists, architects, and otherwise interested individuals began proposing alternative resting places for the dead. Along with changes in burial practices discussed in chapters 2 and 3, many people before and after the Revolution championed changes in nomenclature and landscape design, preferring terms like *Champs de repos*, *Elysée*, and *Champs-Elysées*, rather than *cimetière* or *charnier*. Scholars have interpreted this shift in attitudes as indicative of a new sensibility that emphasized the soothing effect that burial spaces ought to have to lessen the fear of death among the population.[69] As Pierre Dolivier, the author of a cemetery reform essay, explained in 1800, "Instead of seeing a field of devastation and horror, one should find the image of an Elysium: here a grove, here a small meadow, further on a stream, [or a] bed of flowers

scattered about . . . everywhere, prospects and objects that favor meditation and inspire a feeling of sweet melancholy."[70]

Père Lachaise and other cemeteries throughout the world such as
Mt. Auburn in Massachusetts similarly heeded the Enlightenment-era demand for pastoral cemeteries, but Lenoir developed his Elysium in the
years before any of these institutions opened their gates. If he was following any precedent it was probably Rousseau's landscaped burial place in
Ermenonville, forty kilometers northeast of Paris.[71] Like Ermenonville,
the Elysium welcomed artists as well as pilgrims to delight in the somber melancholy and use the space as a source of inspiration. Indeed, by
1813 there were so many artists flocking to the museum's garden that,
according to Lenoir, the caretaker could not complete his yard work.[72]
Like René-Louis de Girardin, Ermenonville's chief designer, Lenoir erected
memorials throughout his garden to commemorate "great men," but unlike Girardin, who only acquired one corpse (Rousseau's, after he died
at Ermenonville), Lenoir made a point of tracking down as many sets of
"great" bones as he could to fill the museum's Elysium.

Throughout 1799 and 1800 Lenoir collected five sets of human remains to add to the two that he had been holding since the early 1790s.
Descartes and his pupil Jacques Rohault had been a part of Lenoir's collection since he removed them from the church of Saint Geneviève during
the Revolution. Lenoir had assumed that Descartes, the "father of French
Philosophy" would be transferred to the Panthéon, but that turned out
not to be the case.[73] In the spring of 1799 Lenoir made his first new acquisition, when he had the mummified remains of general Turenne, which
had been preserved at the Jardin de Plantes since their removal from Saint-
Denis, transferred to the museum's garden. Several months later, in the
autumn of 1799 Lenoir had two seventeenth-century writers, Molière and
La Fontaine, exhumed and transferred from the church of Saint-Joseph
in Montmartre. Also in the autumn of 1799 Lenoir moved two Benedictine monks and scholars, Montfaucon and Mabillon, from Saint-Germain
abbey to the museum. In the winter of 1800 Boileau, a seventeenth-century
poet and contemporary of Molière and La Fontaine, was reunited with
his contemporaries and friends in the garden. Finally, in the spring of
1800 Lenoir traveled to nearby Nogent-sur-Seine to collect his final (and
favorite) set of human remains: the twelfth-century bones of the famously
ill-fated lovers and philosophers Abélard and Héloïse.

The aesthetic and logic governing the garden contrasted sharply with the museum's interior. Unlike the century rooms, which followed a strict chronology, the tombs, mausoleums, cenotaphs, and urns in the Elysium were scattered throughout the small garden without any explicit order. Lenoir commissioned these burial structures for each of the garden's new inhabitants, but in contrast to the museum's aesthetic, he made few attempts to make them historically accurate in their design. Instead of using them to illustrate the artistic (or political) sensibilities of their age, Lenoir wanted to celebrate and commemorate the residents of his Elysium for their individual accomplishments and interests. Stone griffins propped up Descartes's remains, and la Fontaine's tomb was a simple stone sarcophagus inscribed with animals and scenes from his fables. More dramatically, Bernard de Montfaucon, one of the founders of archaeology and paleography in the eighteenth century, lay beneath an elaborate tomb constructed out of Egyptian figures, hieroglyphs, and some debris dating back to the early medieval period, in homage to his antiquarian interests.[74] The order and "authenticity" that governed the museum's interior gave way to deliberate anachronism in the garden. In this respect, the museum and its garden could not have been more different: The museum was organized around the principle of change over time, while the garden exemplified "timeless" virtues, like genius, love, and friendship.

The only garden tomb that Lenoir made as historically accurate as possible was the elaborate monument he built for Abélard and Héloïse. He enclosed their bones together in the tomb that had been originally built for Abélard by one of his colleagues in the twelfth century and surrounded the tomb with a sepulchral chapel built out of debris from various medieval structures. Lenoir went out of his way to construct an "authentic" funeral monument for their seven-hundred-year-old bones.[75] He also wanted their recumbent *gisants*, which topped their tombs, to be accurate representations of their likeness, unlike the "ridiculous" medallions of the two in Notre Dame, which featured anachronistic hairstyles and clothing.[76] Part of the reason certainly had to do with the popularity of the lovers' story. The monument dedicated to Abélard and Héloïse was easily the most popular attraction at the museum. Even before the tragic couple arrived at Petits-Augustins, Parisians were showing up at the museum hoping to see them.[77] In a mildly critical description of the museum, one British travel writer noted how "crowds of persons of all descriptions, who pass unheeded by sovereigns, wits, statesmen, and heroes, pause instinctively before that of Abélard."[78] Lenoir acknowledged that the public's interest in Abélard and Héloïse probably reflected a macabre attraction to stories of suffering and unhappiness rather than an appreciation for medieval philosophy, but far from playing down the significance of the couple's tragic story he emphasized it, with an eye to pointing out the cruelty of the medieval church.[79] Lenoir believed that by paying homage to the two medieval lovers he was undoing the work of an era, "plunged into the shadows of superstition."[80] In his published description of the tomb, Lenoir quoted passages from their letters that critiqued the "ruthless regulations" of monastic life.[81] To encase the lovers in a medieval-looking monument was to continually remind visitors how closely their unhappiness was bound to the "barbarity" of their age and the clerical institutions that destroyed them.

This subtle anticlericalism was also evident in the inclusion of the highly symbolic, but empty tomb of Gaspard de Coligny in the garden. Coligny had been the leader of the French Huguenots before he met a dramatic end in 1572 during the St. Bartholomew's Day Massacre, in which thousands of Huguenots were slaughtered in one of France's bloodiest acts of religious violence. Coligny was shot in the street and subsequently defenestrated and decapitated. His remains were secretly stolen away by his friends and hid in the basement of a castle for over two hundred years. In 1786 a private individual built a small chapel and sarcophagus to contain Coligny's remains in the middle of a lush green space beside a river surrounded by weeping willows and cypress trees. The monument was inscribed with verses from Voltaire, who had written about the death of Coligny earlier in the century in his *Henriade,* touting Coligny's courage in the face of death and recounting the gruesome fate of his corpse.[82] When the property containing the tomb was sold during the Revolution, Lenoir decided to rescue the funeral monument and reconstruct it in his garden. "Oh what bitter and delicious memories this monument will foster in the heart of a virtuous man!" He exclaimed, "What sublime reflections for the philosopher!"[83] Lenoir did eventually acquire the tomb but was not before someone absconded with the physical remains of Coligny in year V (1796–97).

One would assume that Lenoir, who never flinched during the exhuming and destruction of the royal tombs at Saint-Denis, would take the disappearance of Coligny's bones in stride. He did, after all, acquire the tomb, which he considered a valuable artistic contribution to the museum's collection. However, the published description of the tomb reveals how distressed Lenoir was over the loss of Coligny's remains. He inveighed against the "cowardly thief" who raided Coligny's grave: "For all people, in all times, respect for the dead is a virtue, and the violation of tombs is a crime . . . well! insolent despoiler, whoever you are, I call down upon you the infamy of the entire earth and of all centuries, I condemn your soul to the furies!"[84] By 1805 when Lenoir published this, his museum contained hundreds of tombs that had probably been emptied within the previous ten years, yet this four-page tirade against the violation of Coligny's grave stands out in his writing as the only time that he appeared troubled by the absence of a corpse.

Lenoir's anger over Coligny's stolen bones highlights the critical difference between the museum and its garden. Empty tombs suited the interior of the museum where the tombs themselves represented stages in the nation's art and history. Moreover, their emptiness was the thing that made them acceptable in a postrevolutionary environment, since they continually recalled the destruction of hereditary monarchy while illustrating its history. By contrast, the individuals contained in the garden posed no threat to the postrevolutionary regime's legitimacy; instead they represented values and narratives that remained relevant for the nineteenth century. Lenoir wanted Coligny's remains in his garden because he thought that his death called out for religious toleration—an ostensible hallmark of the postrevolutionary era. However, Lenoir's description of how Coligny's remains were secretly commemorated and maintained throughout the eighteenth century also made him into a great symbol of fraternal devotion and love. And love, both romantic and fraternal, was one of the key values that Lenoir sought to promote in his garden.

Abélard and Héloïse's tomb was certainly Lenoir's most celebrated monument to love. By the nineteenth century, the history of the two lovers' remains had become almost as legendary as their lives: after their deaths in the twelfth century the remains of the forcibly estranged lovers were secretly reunited and kept in close proximity to one another. By 1780 they had even begun sharing a (divided) coffin. Lenoir took possession of their remains in 1801, but it was not until he finally completed their elaborate sepulchral chapel in 1807 that he fulfilled a 750-year-old mission by mingling their bones together. "Set deep in their tomb," he wrote, "these inseparable friends live again."[85] Henry Redhead Yorke similarly imagined "the sighs of tenderness and love" escaping from the tomb and echoing throughout the garden as the two medieval lovers called out to one another.[86] Lenoir once described this project as "animated by the ardor of love and by the fire of genius"—quite a stretch from the chilly and dispassionate history on display inside of the museum.[87]

Lenoir invoked a similar duty to friendship when he pursued the remains of the seventeenth-century writers Molière and La Fontaine. He justified the acquisition not by appealing to artistic merit or impending destruction (indeed, both tombs were being kept safely in a church in Montmartre). Rather, he offered his garden as the perfect resting place to mount a monument dedicated to both "French literature and friendship." He proposed a plan to place the remains in a sarcophagus next to a monument featuring busts of Molière, Boileau, la Fontaine, and Racine.[88] His request was approved, and one month later, on May 5, 1800, he collected the remains of the two famous seventeenth-century writers, brought them back to the museum, and deposited their bones in newly constructed tombs beside a path on a small green hill spotted with pansies, violets, and myrtle.[89] Boileau's remains were enclosed in a nearby tomb the following spring.[90] True to his word, Lenoir erected a small "monument to friendship" that featured the busts of the four writers (although Racine's remains were never transferred to the museum). Self-impressed, Lenoir noted how during their lifetime "a gentle friendship often brought these illustrious men together. . . . A religious sentiment reunited them in our Elysium."[91]

Significantly, when Lenoir invoked "religious sentiment," it was explicitly secular. This struck some contemporaries as odd and off-putting, given his adoption of the quasi-religious term *elysée* for his garden. In his published description of the Elysium, however, Lenoir addressed this directly by systematically historicizing the concept of the Elysium, dating back to ancient Egypt. At all times and in all cultures, he explained, one finds binary depictions of a positive (*elysée*) and negative (*tartar*) afterlife, that reflect the values and collective imagination of the society that invented them. However, Lenoir continued, if an *elysée* actually existed as a reward for a virtuous life, the only place one might locate it was in the satisfying sentiment of having treated his fellows well, and the desire to continue such behavior in the future. Inspired in no small measure by Condorcet's famous *Esquisse*, Lenoir explained that the "true Elysium" had nothing to do with a heavenly afterlife; rather, it could be found in the awareness of one's positive contribution to the world in which they lived.[92] Men like Molière and La Fontaine certainly improved their world by making it more beautiful with their work, but their monument in the Elysian Garden also emphasized the inspiring art of friendship.

Friendship in the age of the Revolution has been slowly gaining momentum among scholars.[93] Particularly in the aftermath of the Terror, when the social order was in flux and bonds of trust buckled at all levels of society, the "religion" of friendship offered an appealing avenue to social cohesion. This regularly played out between the tombstones at Père Lachaise, as chapter 4 demonstrated, so perhaps it should not be surprising that it also appeared in the Museum of French Monuments' backyard cemetery. While Lenoir wanted museum visitors to comprehend the history of France before the Revolution as a clear process of development and decline, the Elysian Garden celebrated the social bond of friendship. In this way, the Museum of French Monuments became an unlikely space of reunion and concord in the early nineteenth century. Lenoir applauded himself for reuniting Abélard and Héloïse, or La Fontaine, Molière, and Boileau not only with each other, but also with the city of Paris, to which he believed they "belonged."[94] Thus, despite all of the hard work that Lenoir had done to thwart and undo the "vandalism" of the Terror, he was delighted when a guest to the garden engraved an impromptu epitaph on La Fontaine's tomb and he fondly boasted about how "lovers wanted to inscribe their names on the tomb of Héloïse and Abélard."[95] As Louis Courajod, the nineteenth-century director of the Louvre, explained it, Lenoir's work had "precipitated the work of time" by bringing together the living and the dead.[96]

It is ubiquitous in history for new regimes to destroy significant monuments from the past. This was especially the case during the French Revolution, when radicals invented, only to destroy, the "Old Regime" and sought to obliterate as many traces of the past as possible. But, of course, such aggressive presentism also gave rise to a conservationist movement and by the beginning of the nineteenth century, France was experiencing a complex and often contradictory relationship with its past, both distant and recent. The Museum of French Monuments was born out of these contrasting impulses, and as this chapter has argued the dead were essential to negotiating that tension. Inside the museum, their conspicuous absence made the distant past acceptable while providing opportunities to reflect on the recent violence of the Terror. Outside in the garden, paeans to buried "geniuses" offered models for socially cohesive behavior moving forward. In both cases, the meticulous ordering of the dead—or their tombs—was at the heart of the museum's ability to function as a soothing escape from the tumult and dislocation of the era. After a visit in February 1800, one Frenchman wrote to Lenoir to thank him for constructing such an effective "refuge of contemplation and tranquility." He elaborated, "Those of us who are extremely exhausted by the violent blows of the raging storm find a guaranteed respite in the restoration that you provide." The use of the word *restauration* may have had a double meaning in this case: just as Lenoir restored historic monuments, so too did the "fine order of things" at the museum act as a restorative balm for weary visitors.[97]

It should come as no surprise that the Museum of French Monuments did not survive the political Restoration of the Bourbon monarchy, which gradually but permanently disestablished the museum between 1814 and 1816. On August 30, the new king Louis XVIII ordered Lenoir to relinquish a large part of the museum's property to a neighboring institution. Significantly, the revoked territory included the apartments of the museum's employees and a large part of the museum's garden. This confiscation foreshadowed tougher days ahead and as members of the old aristocracy began to slowly filter back into Paris, they returned to the Museum of French Monuments to collect their confiscated belongings.[98] On April 24, 1816, after the second Restoration, a royal proclamation effectively dissolved the museum by legally restoring the monuments to their prior owners and by the end of that year the museum officially closed its doors for good. For the next three years churches and returning émigrés reclaimed their property, the entombed "geniuses" made their way to Père Lachaise Cemetery, and Lenoir returned the royal tombs to Saint-Denis where they remain to this day.

CONCLUSION

The Historian of the Dead

At its most basic this book has told the story of how the cemetery transformed in Paris, from a space of danger to a site for social reconstruction and reinvention. By the end of the Old Regime, the dead were increasingly understood as a menace to public health in the capital, and ancient burial sites, like the Cemetery of the Innocents, were being razed to the ground. At this crucial moment when the place and meaning of the dead in the city were under negotiation, the Revolution intervened and violently changed the terms of debate. On one hand, the revolutionaries redeemed the dead and their spaces by placing them at the center of a cultural project of moral, social, and civic regeneration. However, the miserable state of revolutionary cemeteries coupled with the terrifying spectacle of thousands of headless corpses ultimately produced an even more urgent crisis. By the end of the Terror in 1794, Parisians viewed the dead in their city as both a hygienic emergency and a brutal reminder of revolutionary failure.

Perhaps this was why decades later, one of the nineteenth century's most evocative historians of the Revolution accented his account of the frenetic summer of 1794 with a vivid description of Parisian cemeteries. Toward the end of the seventh and last volume of his *Histoire de la révolution française*, Jules Michelet used spaces for the dead as both material and symbolic evidence of the Revolution's failure. He explained how in Picpus Cemetery, the dense ground had begun to expel headless corpses, in seeming defiance of the Jacobins' attempt to bury their victims. "The clay rejected it all," he wrote, "it refused to hide anything. Everything returned to the surface. Liquid putrefaction bubbled in the hot summer sun."[1] This rich sensory description reflects the language of the archival sources in which Michelet immersed himself, but it also demonstrates how, even fifty years after their dissolution, the cemeteries of the Terror effectively represented the very worst that the Revolution had to offer. If a revolutionary population could not be trusted to respectfully honor their dead—the most "natural" of human impulses—how could they possibly hope to remake the world?

A good place to start, as it turned out, was in the cemetery. As this book has demonstrated, commentary about Parisian cemeteries in the wake of the Terror was about more than civil reform; it also revealed much deeper anxieties about the consequences and legacies of the Revolution. Chief among these was the overwhelming and perennially incomplete task of reimagining (and eventually reforming) the social world. Revolutionaries successfully demolished France's longstanding social order premised on privilege and promised to replace it with a more just system of organization based on Enlightenment principles like equality and fraternity. This audacious task inspired the revolutionary population with both excitement about the possibilities of regeneration and fear about impending social collapse, especially after the suspicion and violence of the Terror. Michelet aptly captured this tension in his description of the infamous *Bal des Zéphirs* of 1794, at which young Parisians were rumored to have danced atop tombstones. Rather than reading these dances as acts of "impious frivolity" that signaled social breakdown, he proposed a rosier view, suggesting that if the dead were to have reawakened during these macabre festivities, "they would have been happy to witness this rebirth of society" after the trauma of the Terror.[2] However, Michelet's generous reading of these notorious dances came seven full decades after their occurrence. In 1794, this initial release of exhilaration was overshadowed by uncertainty and anxiety about the form that this "reborn" society should take.

Spaces for the dead—both imagined and enacted—quickly emerged after 1794 as venues where many of these social anxieties could be expressed, contemplated, and possibly even resolved. Just as the oozing mass graves of the Terror offered an analogy of chaos, so too did the tree-lined boulevards of Père Lachaise, the bone-filled tunnels of the Catacombs, and the chronologically organized tombs in the Museum of French Monuments provide soothing images of restored order. What this "order" looked like varied significantly, from radical egalitarianism to hierarchies of wealth and merit, which only demonstrates how expansive the legacy of the Revolution was becoming. In addition to supplying these images of order, spaces for the dead also created opportunities for cohesion and connection, by uniting disparate groups of Parisians with each other, with their city, and with their shared past. These sites certainly had their detractors who railed against them for being too homogenizing, too ostentatious, or too academic, but they also had multitudes of devotees who flocked to their gates, eager to enter the city, empire, and museum of the dead.

Jules Michelet is possibly the best known of these nineteenth-century cemetery enthusiasts. Although he had been to Père Lachaise earlier in his life, it was not until the death of his best friend, Paul Poinsot, in February 1821 that Michelet began making regular visits to the "city of the dead" as he would later call it.[3] A week after Poinsot's death, Michelet made a solemn declaration in his private journal that henceforth "Père Lachaise will be my *lieu de prédilection*." He found the cemetery to be aesthetically pleasing, but also calming to his soul, which was wracked by the loss of his companion. In Père Lachaise, a liminal space that Michelet described as sitting "between earth and heaven," he and Poinsot could "continue to live together."[4] Subsequent journal entries reveal that the young historian meant what he wrote: he returned to Poinsot's grave almost daily for weeks, sometimes accompanied by friends and family, other times he just brought manuscripts-in-progress, which he wanted to edit in the presence of his dead friend.[5] Even after his attachment to Poinsot faded, Michelet continued making regular trips to the cemetery. These visits always included outpourings of emotion and small acts of communion at the graves of friends and heroes, such as the liberal political thinker Benjamin Constant, whose "neglected" grave Michelet visited for years.[6]

Michelet's connection to the cemetery also extended beyond the personal. Like many of the subjects who appeared in chapters 3, 4, and 5 of this book, he used Père Lachaise to connect with his fellow Parisians as well as with the city he loved. He regularly reflected on the tombstones of strangers, sometimes recording particularly evocative burial sites in his journal, such as that of a young mother who shared a tomb with her five-year-old daughter.[7] Since his youth he had always been particularly struck by so-called "neglected" graves and took care to tend to them, whenever possible.[8] However, while he often singled out specific graves for attention, Michelet's lifelong devotion was to the cemetery as a whole. He first declared this commitment in September 1820, when he visited the tomb of his childhood friend, Sophie. After spending an entire afternoon in the peaceful environment of the cemetery, the twenty-two-year-old Michelet had something of an epiphany. He looked around him and felt an overwhelming sense of sympathy for the Parisians beneath his feet. "Poor Sophie! Poor dead people! I will return to see you," he promised. "From this tomb," he announced, "I will think about Paris and invite her to rest after this long and arduous journey called life."[9]

Fourteen years later, when reflecting back on his early adulthood, Michelet made explicit the link between himself, the cemetery, and the city he loved. "If I decide, sooner or later (and it will be later) to summarize the memories of my individual existence," he wrote, "I shall take as its center, its text, its theatre, Père Lachaise cemetery."[10] In "this admirable theatre of life and death . . . the individual passions of a young man seem less small. . . . His personal passions borrow something grand and philosophical from the contrasts of a site that is simultaneously so charming and so tragic."[11] This statement reveals more than Michelet's macabre obsession with the cemetery: a century and a half before Foucault, Michelet understood the cemetery as a kind of heterotopia. He marveled at its ability to hold in balance so many opposite conditions and understood this ability as the source of its power. In addition to life/death and charm/tragedy, he also noted silence/birdsong; solemn tombs/vibrant roses; and grief/love. For Michelet, this Otherness led to a strange alchemy by which he was able to unite his individual self with the collective people of Paris; the same phenomena observed in the Catacombs in chapter 4. And like visitors to the Catacombs, Michelet took advantage of this process to glean an intimate understanding of his city's history. Indeed, six weeks before making this declaration, he explained how it was "from this city of the dead facing the city of the living" that he finally understood the history of his age. By switching his gaze between monuments in the city below him and the monuments to the dead in the cemetery, he observed three distinct epochs (the Empire, Restoration, and July Monarchy) inhabiting the same space.[12] Significantly, when he made that observation he was in the early months of his life's work: writing a comprehensive history of France, a project that would consume him for the next forty years.[13]

Père Lachaise Cemetery was not the only space for the dead that inspired Michelet's sense of history. As noted briefly in chapter 5, he also had strong and positive childhood recollections of ambling through the halls of the Museum of French Monuments. In 1840 he told Alfred Dumesnil, his pupil and future son-in-law, that he had been "practically raised" in Lenoir's museum and that it had "singularly influenced" his ideas about history.[14] Like Père Lachaise, the Museum of French Monuments "revealed" the history of France to a young Michelet by bringing together the dead in a sublime and powerful order. In the museum, he wrote, "national perpetuity was reproduced. One could finally see France as she was, in her development, from century to century and from man to man, from tomb to tomb."[15] Despite its studied chronology, the museum in Michelet's view effectively brought the different epochs of France's history into conversation with one another, because "the entombed dead render[ed] all times contemporaries."[16] As Michelet experienced and remembered it, the museum made the expansive past legible by containing it all in place, but this process only worked because of the cohesive power of the dead.

Surprisingly, considering his attachment to Paris's macabre sites, no record exists of young Michelet having toured the Catacombs. However, "Catacombs" appear as a vivid metaphor in the third volume of his *History of France* when recounting his first experience in the National Archives. In October 1830 the minister of the interior (François Guizot) appointed Michelet as the head of the historical section of the National Archives. As Michelet later described it, "These manuscript catacombs . . . this necropolis of national monuments" immediately struck him as alive with meaning and potential. He continued,

These papers, these long-forgotten parchments only asked to be rediscovered. These papers were not papers, but the lives of men, of provinces, of peoples. Families and fiefs, emblazoned in their dust, protested against oblivion. . . . All lived and spoke, they surrounded me with an army of a thousand languages which together formed the voice of the Republic and the Empire.[17]

Michelet was the first scholar to write the history of France using these archives, but he understood this work in ways that are almost incomprehensible to twenty-first-century scholars.[18] In Michelet's archive, the past rushed forth through dusty texts—the bones of his "manuscript catacombs"—and demanded to be heard. He met this demand by writing some of the most detailed and affecting accounts of French history, a process he alternately described as an act of exhumation, resurrection, and communion.[19] The version of France that emerged in these histories always placed "the people" at its heart, with fraternal love as its stabilizing and uniting force.[20]

In his famous takedown of Revolutionary historiography, François Furet used Michelet as an example of what not to do. Placing him in opposition to the more analytical Tocqueville, Furet described Michelet as someone who "brings the Revolution back to life from the inside" by commemorating and communing with the past. In Furet's assessment, this approach blinded the historian to the "gulf between the Revolution's true outcome and the revolutionaries' intentions."[21] However, in the context of the postrevolutionary city, Michelet's methodology reveals a remarkable triumph. In the aftermath of a Revolution that declared war on the past followed by a royal Restoration that in turn swore to "forget" the Revolution, Michelet demonstrated an uncanny ability to make sense of his nation's long and fraught history. As this conclusion has demonstrated, he developed this uniquely personal approach to studying the past while spending hours in the midst of Paris's dead. In Père Lachaise, and the Museum of French Monuments before it, Michelet learned to link his individual self to "the general" consciousness of his city, which made it possible for him to then "resurrect" its history.

Michelet was hardly your average nineteenth-century Parisian, but his life and work vividly illuminate the significance and power of spaces for the dead in the postrevolutionary era. These sites bore no resemblance to the fetid pits of the Old Regime and Revolution, but neither were they the tightly organized didactic spaces that reformers dreamed up in the

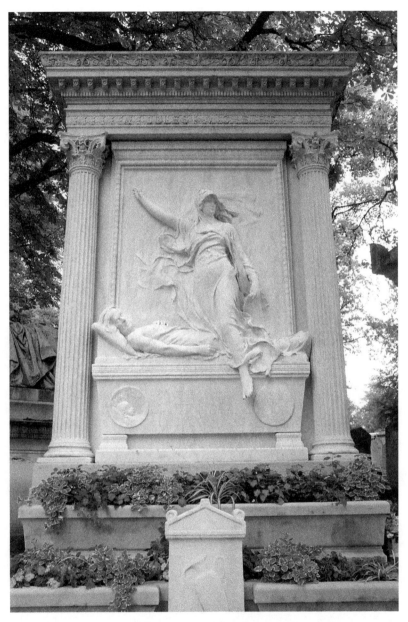

Figure C.1. The tomb of Jules Michelet in Père Lachaise Cemetery.
Author's photograph.

1790s. Instead, they developed as quietly unifying spaces whose aesthetics and organization offered alternate models for a reimagined social world, whether as a hierarchy of wealth and virtue that recognized individual accomplishments or as an egalitarian celebration of collective identity. Underpinning both of these alternatives, however, was an understanding that a shared history—on a personal, citywide, and national level—was essential to holding this new world together. And when Michelet claimed to resurrect the past by haunting the alleys of Père Lachaise Cemetery, he demonstrated how central spaces for the dead were to this process. At the threshold that linked the living to the dead, Parisians embraced their past in order to understand the present, and prepare for the future.

NOTES

Introduction: The Revolution of the Dead

1. The first collection of bones was transferred into the Catacombs four months after the excavations began, on April 7, 1786.

2. Louis-Sébastien Mercier, *Tableau de Paris*, vol. 9 (Amsterdam, 1783–89), 192–93.

3. C.-P. Arnaud, *Receuil de tombeaux des quatre cimetières de Paris, avec leurs epitaphs et leurs inscriptions*, vol. 1 (Paris: Arnaud, 1817), 81, 85, 91.

4. Jules Michelet, *Histoire de la Révolution française*, 2nd ed. (Paris: Librairie internationale, 1869), 10:297.

5. Thomas Détruisard, *Essai sur les Catacombes de Paris* (Paris, 1812), 18.

6. Mona Ozouf even notes that "it was in the funerary festivals that the most determined expressionism of the Revolutionary festival was to survive." *Festivals and the French Revolution*, trans. Alan Sheridan (Cambridge, MA: Harvard University Press, 1988), 81.

7. Jean-Baptiste Avril, *Rapport de l'administration des travaux publics, sur les cimetières* (Paris, 1794), 1–2, 18, 20.

8. The four most influential texts about the history of death in the West from this era are Philippe Ariès, *The Hour of Our Death*, trans. Helen Weaver (New York: Knopf, 1981); Michel Vovelle, *Le Mort et l'Occident de 1300 à nos jours* (Paris: Gallimard, 1983); Pierre Chaunu, *La Mort à Paris 16e, 17e, 18e siècles* (Paris: Fayard, 1978); John McManners, *Death and the Enlightenment: Changing Attitudes to Death among Christians and Unbelievers in*

Eighteenth-century France (Oxford: Oxford University Press, 1981). Ariès's comment about being an "Anarchist of the right" appears several times in Patrick H. Hutton's *Philippe Ariès and the Politics of French Cultural History* (Amherst: University of Massachusetts Press, 2004).

9. Craig Koslofsky, *The Reformation of the Dead: Death and Ritual in Early Modern Germany, 1450–1700* (New York: St. Martin's Press, 2000); Vanessa Harding, *The Dead and the Living in Paris and London, 1500–1670* (Cambridge: Cambridge University Press, 2002); Thomas Laqueur, *The Work of the Dead: A Cultural History of Mortal Remains* (Princeton, NJ: Princeton University Press, 2015).

10. Laqueur, *The Work of the Dead*, 13.

11. Antoine de Baecque, *Glory and Terror: Seven Deaths under the French Revolution*, trans. Charlotte Mandell (New York: Routledge, 2001), 8.

12. Colin Lucas, "Revolutionary Violence," in *The French Revolution and the Creation of Modern Political Culture*, ed. Keith Michael Baker, vol. 4, *The Terror* (Oxford: Pergamon Press, 1994), 57–79.

13. Joseph Clarke, *Commemorating the Dead in Revolutionary France: Revolution and Remembrance, 1789–1799* (Cambridge: Cambridge University Press, 2007). Other books that emphasize the political power of funerals in nineteenth-century France include Avner Ben-Amos, *Funerals, Politics, and Memory in Modern France, 1789–1996* (Oxford: Oxford University Press, 2000); and Patrick H. Hutton, *The Cult of the Revolutionary Tradition: The Blanquists in French Politics, 1864–1893* (Berkeley: University of California Press, 1981). On the Panthéon specifically, see Jean-Claude Bonnet, *Naissance du Panthéon: Essai sur le culte des grands hommes* (Paris: Fayard, 1998); Mona Ozouf, "Le Panthéon: L'école normale des morts," in *Les lieux de mémoire*, ed. Pierre Nora (Paris: Gallimard, 1984), 1:139–66; and Annie Jourdan, *Les Monuments de la Révolution, 1770–1804: Une histoire de représentation* (Paris: Champion, 1997).

14. Richard Etlin explores these ideas in intricate detail in *The Architecture of Death: The Transformation of the Cemetery in Eighteenth-Century Paris* (Cambridge, MA: MIT Press, 1984) and to a lesser extent in *Symbolic Space: French Enlightenment Architecture and Its Legacy* (Chicago: University of Chicago Press, 1994).

15. Emmanuel Fureix, *La France des larmes: deuils politiques à l'âge romantique, 1814–1840* (Seyssel: Champ Vallon, 2009).

16. Bronislaw Baczko, *Ending the Terror: The French Revolution after Robespierre*, trans. Michel Petheram (Cambridge: Cambridge University Press, 1994); Ronald Schechter, "Gothic Thermidor: The Bals des victimes, the Fantastic, and the Production of Historical Knowledge in Post-Terror France," *Representations* 61 (winter 1998): 78–94; Joseph Zizek, "'Plum de Fer': Louis-Marie Prudhomme Writes the French Revolution," *French Historical Studies* 26, no. 4 (fall 2003): 619–60; Howard Brown, *Ending the Revolution: Violence, Justice, and Repression from the Terror to Napoleon* (Charlottesville: University of Virginia Press, 2006); Ronen Steinberg, "Trauma and the Effects of Mass Violence in Revolutionary France: A Critical Inquiry," *Historical Reflections* 41, no. 3 (December 2015): 28–46; Ronen Steinberg, "Terror on Trial: Accountability, Transitional Justice, and the *Affair Le Bon* in Thermidorian France," *French Historical Studies* 39, no. 3 (August 2016): 419–44; Laura Mason, "The Culture of Reaction: Demobilizing the People after Thermidor," *French Historical Studies* 39, no. 3 (August 2016): 445–70. Moreover, *French Historical Studies* has dedicated two fora to the theme of "Thermidor and the French Revolution," in 38, no. 1 (February 2015) and 39, no. 3 (August 2016).

17. Denise Z. Davidson, *France after Revolution: Urban Life, Gender, and the New Social Order* (Cambridge, MA: Harvard University Press, 2007). Davidson makes a convincing case for considering the Empire and Restoration together as a single "postrevolutionary"

era, characterized by the project to "build a stable political and social order that would survive despite the post-1789 recognition that governments, if unpopular or unsuccessful, could be toppled" (8).

18. Isser Woloch, *The New Regime: Transformations in the French Civic Order, 1789–1820s* (New York: W. W. Norton, 1994); Ralph Kingston, *Bureaucrats and Bourgeois Society: Office Politics and Individual Credit in France, 1789–1848* (New York: Palgrave Macmillan, 2012); Sarah Maza, *The Myth of the French Bourgeoisie: An Essay on the Social Imaginary* (Cambridge, MA: Harvard University Press, 2003); Rebecca Spang, *The Invention of the Restaurant: Paris and Modern Gastronomic Culture* (Cambridge, MA: Harvard University Press, 2000); Jan Goldstein, *The Post-Revolutionary Self: Politics and Psyche in France, 1750–1850* (Cambridge, MA: Harvard University Press, 2005).

19. Laura Mason, "Never Was a Plot So Holy: Gracchus Babeuf and the End of the French Revolution," in *Conspiracy and the French Revolution*, ed. Thomas Kaiser, Marisa Linton, and Peter Campbell (Manchester: Manchester University Press, 2007), 172–88; Andrew Jainchill, *Reimagining Politics after the Terror: The Republican Origins of French Liberalism* (Ithaca, NY: Cornell University Press, 2008); Carolina Armenteros, *The French Idea of History: Joseph de Maistre and His Heirs, 1794–1854* (Ithaca, NY: Cornell University Press, 2011).

20. Henri Lefebvre, *The Production of Space*, trans. Donald Nicholson-Smith (Oxford: Wiley-Blackwell, 1991), 59.

21. Victoria Thompson, "Telling 'Spatial Stories': Urban Space and Bourgeois Identity in Early Nineteenth-Century Paris," *Journal of Modern History* 75, no. 3 (September 2003): 530, 534.

22. Dominique Kalifa, "Crime Scenes: Criminal Topography and Social Imaginary in Nineteenth-Century Paris," trans. Martine Andreoli, *French Historical Studies* 27, no. 1 (winter 2004): 176.

23. Alain Corbin, *The Foul and the Fragrant: Odor and the French Social Imagination* (Cambridge, MA: Harvard University Press, 1988), 5. For more on foul smells and the social order in (late) nineteenth-century France, see David S. Barnes, *The Great Stink of Paris and the Nineteenth-Century Struggle against Filth and Germs* (Baltimore: Johns Hopkins University Press, 2006). For an interdisciplinary and transnational approach, see William A. Cohen and Ryan Johnson, eds., *Filth: Dirt, Disgust, and Modern Life* (Minneapolis: University of Minnesota Press, 2005).

24. Michel Ragon, *The Space of Death: A Study of Funerary Architecture, Decoration, and Urbanism* (Charlottesville: University Press of Virginia, 1983), 19.

25. Specifically, Turner writes that "it is the analysis of culture into factors and their free recombination in any and every possible pattern, however weird, that is most characteristic of liminality." Victor Turner, *Dramas, Fields, and Metaphors: Symbolic Action in Human Society* (Ithaca, NY: Cornell University Press, 1974), 255.

26. The first published version of this essay appeared in the October 1984 issue of the French journal *Architecture-Mouvement-Continuité*. It was based on a public lecture that Foucault gave in March 1967. The English translation appeared two years later as Michel Foucault, "Of Other Spaces," trans. Jay Miskowiec, *Diacritics: A Review of Contemporary Criticism* 16, no. 1 (spring 1986): 22–27. The discussion of the cemetery as a "strange Heterotopia" occurs on page 25.

27. Foucault, "Of Other Spaces," 25.

28. Ibid., 26.

29. Two recent works have tackled the previously understudied revolutionary calendar: Matthew Shaw, *Time and the French Revolution: The Republican Calendar, 1789–Year XIV* (London: Boydell Press, 2011); and Sanja Perovic, *The Calendar in Revolutionary France: Perceptions of Time in Literature, Culture, Politics* (Cambridge: Cambridge University Press, 2012).

30. Stephen Bann, *Romanticism and the Rise of History* (New York: Twayne, 1995).

31. Reinhart Koselleck, *Future's Past: On the Semantics of Historical Time,* trans. Keith Tribe (New York: Columbia University Press, 1985); Peter Fritzsche, *Stranded in the Present: Modern Time and the Melancholy of History* (Cambridge, MA: Harvard University Press, 2004); Harold Mah, "The French Revolution and the Problem of Time: Hegel to Marx," in *Enlightenment Phantasies: Cultural Identity in France and Germany, 1750–1914* (Ithaca, NY: Cornell University Press, 2003), 157–80.

32. Harding, *The Dead and the Living in Paris and London,* 85.

33. Louis-Sébastien Mercier, "Sur le dépôt des Petits-Augustins, dit: le musée des monuments français," *Journal d'économie publique, de morale, et de politique* 5 (1797): 327–28.

Chapter 1. The Problem of the Dead

1. Antoine-Alexis Cadet de Vaux, "Mémoire historique et physique sur le cimetière des Innocents," *Journal de Physique* (June 1783): 410–11, 416–17.

2. John McManners, *Death and the Enlightenment: Changing Attitudes to Death among Christians and Unbelievers in Eighteenth-century France* (Oxford: Oxford University Press, 1981).

3. For more on the Panthéon and the Revolution, see Barry Bergdoll, ed., *Le Panthéon: Symbole des révolutions* (Paris: Picard, 1989); and Joseph Clarke, *Commemorating the Dead in Revolutionary France, 1789–1799* (Cambridge: Cambridge University Press, 2007), especially chapter 3, "The Founding Fathers of Liberty," 87–126. For a comparative approach, see Richard Wrigley and Matthew Kraske, eds., *Pantheons: Transformations of a Monumental Idea* (London: Ashgate, 2004); and Eveline Bouwers, *Public Pantheons in Revolutionary Europe: Comparing Cultures, c. 1790–1840* (New York: Palgrave, 2012). On the process of constructing the Panthéon, see Alan Potofsky, *Constructing Paris in the Age of Revolution* (London: Palgrave Macmillan, 2009), 105–11.

4. Other than Clarke, cited above, who focuses on the politics of commemoration during the Revolutionary era, see Avner Ben-Amos, *Funerals, Politics, and Memory in Modern France, 1789–1996* (Oxford: Oxford University Press, 2005), especially chapter 1, "The French Revolution and the Emergence of Republican State Funerals, 1789–1799," 17–53. For analysis of the politics of the corpse during the Revolution, see Antoine de Baecque, *Glory and Terror: Seven Deaths under the French Revolution,* trans. Charlotte Mandel (New York: Routledge, 2001). Much has been written about revolutionary violence in the last decade. Notable titles include Jean-Clément Martin, *Violence et Révolution: Essai sur la naissance d'un mythe national* (Paris: Éditions de Seuil, 2006); Sophie Wahnich, *In Defense of the Terror: Liberty or Death in the French Revolution,* trans. David Fernbach (New York: Verso, 2012); Micah Alpaugh, *Non-violence and the French Revolution: Political Demonstrations in Paris, 1787–1795* (Cambridge: Cambridge University Press, 2015).

5. This number is based on the 1763 report from the Châtelet Officers about the state of Parisian cemeteries. It includes thirty churchyard cemeteries as well as the cemetery for L'Hôpital de la charité and for the Collège du Cardinal Lemoine. BNF Joly de Fleury 1209, "Avis des Officiers du Châtelet au sujet des cimetières," 10–25.

6. Madeleine Foisil, "Les attitudes devant la mort aux XVIIIe siècle: sépultures et suppressions de sépultures dans le cimetière Parisien des Saints-Innocents," *Revue Historique* 251 (April–June 1974): 312. This number is significantly lower than the three thousand that Louis-Sébastien Mercier estimated in 1788.

7. Vanessa Harding, *The Dead and the Living in Paris and London, 1500–1670* (Cambridge: Cambridge University Press, 2002), 75, 85, 101, 105. The cemetery was owned jointly by the dean and chapter of Saint-Germain-l'Auxerrois, the Hospital of Sainte-Catherine, and the Hospital of Hôtel-Dieu.

8. Alain Corbin, *The Foul and the Fragrant* (Cambridge, MA: Harvard University Press, 1988), 15–16. Richard Eltlin also describes how scientists like Antoine-Laurent de Lavoisier (a Parisian) visited crowded theaters and hospitals to capture foul-smelling air in beakers to analyze its composition in his laboratory. Richard Etlin, "The Cemetery and the City: Paris, 1744–1804" (Ph.D. diss., Princeton University, 1978), 19.

9. Owen and Caroline Hannaway, "Le fermeture du cimetière des Innocents," *Dix-huitième siècle* 9 (1979): 183–85.

10. BNF, Joly de Fleury 1209, "Avis des officiers du Châtelet au sujet des cimetières," 14.

11. For detailed information about this ordinance and the steps leading up to it, see Jaqueline Thibaut-Payen's impeccably researched administrative history of cemeteries and burial in Old Regime Paris, *Les Morts, l'Église et l'État: Recherches d'histoire administrative sur la sépulture et les cimetières dans le ressort du parlement de Paris aux XVIIe et XVIIIe siècles* (Paris: Fernand Lanore, 1977), 208–26.

12. Quoted in David Garrioch, *The Making of Revolutionary Paris* (Berkeley: University of California Press, 2004), 215.

13. McManners, *Death and the Enlightenment*, 309.

14. Ibid., 314.

15. Cadet de Vaux, "Mémoire historique," 410–11, 416–17.

16. Anon., "Medicine," *Journal de Paris* 279 (October 1781): 1123.

17. Louis-Sébastien Mercier, *Tableau de Paris: Nouvelle édition, corrigée et augmentée*, vol. 9 (Amsterdam, 1788), 325.

18. Ibid., 326.

19. Michel-Augustin Thouret, *Rapport sur les exhumations du cimetière et de l'église des SS Innocents: Lu dans la séance royale de médecine, tenue au Louvre, le 3 mars 1789* (Paris: P.-D. Pierres, 1789), 11. Although Thouret is listed as the author of this report, the document was signed by a committee comprising Geoffroy, Despierres, De Horne, Vicq-D'Azyr, De Fourcroy, and Thouret.

20. Ibid., 14–50.

21. BNF, Joly de Fleury 1209, "A Monseigneur le procureur général, au sujet de ce qu'ils souffrant, des maladies qu'ils éprouvent et du danger au quel ils ont exposés par l'infection et la puanteur du cimetière de la paroisse de St. Eustache, qui par arrangement est aussi celui de celle de St. Germain L'auxerois" (24 August 1786), 107.

22. BNF, Joly de Fleury 1209, "Au monseigneur le procurer général au parlement de Paris," 108–11.

23. Many of these complaints can be found in the Joly de Fleury collection at the Biblio-thèque Nationale de France, cited above.

24. "Séance du mercredi, 11 novembre," *Gazette nationale ou le Moniteur universel* 89 (10–13 November 1789), reprinted in *Réimpression de l'ancien Moniteur,* vol. 2 (Paris: Bureau Central, 1840), 178.

25. Laqueur first made this argument in "The Places of the Dead in Modernity," in *The Age of Cultural Revolutions in Britain and France, 1750–1820,* ed. Colin Jones and Dror Wahrman (Berkeley: University of California Press, 2002), 17–32, and expanded it signif-icantly in *The Work of the Dead: A Cultural History of Mortal Remains* (Princeton, NJ: Princeton University Press, 2015).

26. Desbois de Rochefort, "Lettre au rédacteur," *Gazette nationale ou le Moniteur uni-versel* 162 (11 June 1790), reprinted in *Réimpression de l'ancien Moniteur,* vol. 4 (Paris: Bureau Central, 1841), 591–92.

27. Jessica Goodman, "Introduction," *Commemorating Mirabeau: Mirabeau aux Champs-Elysées and Other Texts,* ed. Jessica Goodman (Cambridge: Modern Humanities Research Association, 2017), 1–52; Clarke, *Revolution and Remembrance in Revolutionary France,* 90–106; de Baecque, *Glory and Terror,* 15–36.

28. Eveline Bouwers, *Public Pantheons in Revolutionary Europe: Comparing Cultures, c. 1790–1840* (New York: Palgrave, 2012).

29. Jean-Louis Vaudoyer, *Idées d'un citoyen sur le lieu destiné à la sépulture des hommes illustres de France* (Paris, 1791), 6.

30. Ibid., 4.

31. Ibid., 7.

32. [Antoine] Quatremère-Quincy, "Politique," *Gazette nationale ou Moniteur universel* 103 (13 April 1791), reprinted in *Réimpression de l'ancien Moniteur*, vol. 8 (Paris: Bureau Centrale, 1841), 109–10.

33. "Séance du Jeudi au soir," *Gazette national, ou le Moniteur universel* 142 (22 May 1791), reprinted in *Réimpression de l'ancien Moniteur*, vol. 8 (Paris: Bureau Centrale, 1841), 456.

34. Charles-Alexandre de Moy, *Accord de la religion et des cultes chez une nation libre* (Paris: J.-B. Garnéry, 1792), 89–94.

35. Ibid., 102.

36. Christine Métayer, "Une espace de vie: Les charniers du cimetière des SS. Innocents à Paris, sous l'Ancien Regime," *Journal of the Canadian Historical Association* 4, no. 1 (1993): 183–206.

37. de Moy, *Accord de la religion et des cultes*, 111.

38. Ibid., 103.

39. Edmond Géraud, *Journal d'un étudiant pendant la Révolution, 1789–1795*, ed. Gaston Maugras (Paris: Calmann Lévy, 1890), 350–51.

40. Brian Singer, "Violence in the French Revolution: Forms of Ingestion/Forms of Expulsion," *Social Research* 56 (spring 1989): 280; David Andress, *The Terror: The Merciless War for Freedom in Revolutionary France* (New York: Farrar, Straus & Giroux, 2005), 114.

41. "Séance du vendredi 7 septembre, à six heurs du soir," *Gazette nationale ou le Moniteur universel* 258 (9 September 1792), reprinted in *Réimpression de l'ancien Moniteur*, vol. 13 (Paris: Bureau Centrale, 1841), 645. Curiously, Bazire's primary concern was not the desecration of tombs and human remains, but the "mephitic vapor" that resulted when these zealous citizens opened ancient tombs to rifle through their contents.

42. "Ode patriotique sur les événemens de l'année 1792, depuis le 10 Août jusqu'au 13 Novembre," in *Odes républicaines au peuple français, composées en Brumaire, l'an IIe, précédées de l'Ode patriotique sur les événemens de l'année 1792* (Paris: Imprimerie nationale des lois, 1795), 9, 17.

43. Louis Prudhomme, *Les Révolutions de Paris*, 29 December 1792–5 January 1793, 83–84.

44. B[ertrand] Barrère, *Rapport fait au nom du comité du salut public, le premier août 1793, l'an II de la république française* (Paris: Imprimerie Nationale, 1793), 28–29.

45. "Notes sur les exhumations de Saint-Denis par un religieux de cette abbaye, témoin oculaire de ces exhumations en 1793," in Le Bon de Guilhermy, *Monographie de l'Église royale de Saint-Denis tombeaux et figures historiques* (Paris, 1848), 55–60.

46. For the eyewitness description that describes the grotto as a "bizarre monument to liberty," see Alexandre Lenoir, "Les tombeaux et les objets d'art de l'église de Saint-Denis," in *Inventaire général des richesses d'art de la France. Archives du Musée des monuments français. Premier partie. Papiers de M. Albert Lenoir et documents tirés des archives de l'administration des beaux-arts* (Paris: Plon, 1883), 15–16. For more analysis of this odd monument, see Erika Naginski, *Sculpture and Enlightenment* (Los Angeles: The Getty Research Institute, 2009), 302–4.

47. Alexandre Lenoir, *Musée des monuments français, ou description historique et chronologique des statues en marbre et en bronze, bas-reliefs et tombeaux des hommes*

et des femmes célèbres, pour servir à l'histoire de France et à celle de L'art, vol. 2 (Paris: Guilleminet, 1801), civ–cv.

48. Suzanne Glover Lindsay has analyzed the royal exhumations of 1793 and notes that "whatever their politics, those present at the exhumations had been conditioned, like many since antiquity, to associate physical corruption with sin even among the living, especially where smells were involved." "The Revolutionary Exhumations at St-Denis, 1793," *Conversations: An Online Journal of the Center for the Study of Material and Visual Cultures of Religion* (2014), doi:10.22332/con.ess.2015.2.

49. For more on the death of Louis XVI and the desacralization of his body, see de Baecque, *Glory and Terror,* 87–119.

50. Georges d'Heilly, *Extraction des cercueils royaux à Saint-Denis en 1793* (Paris: Hachette, 1868), 106.

51. Henriot, "Commune de Paris, séance du 1er frimaire," *Journal de la montagne* 10 (23 November 1793), 75.

52. Anthony Vidler, "The Paradoxes of Vandalism: Henri Grégoire and the Thermidorian Discourse on Historical Monuments," in *The Abbé Grégoire and His World,* ed. Jeremy Popkin and Richard Popkin (Dordrecht: Kluwer, 2000), 129–56.

53. John McManners, *The French Revolution and the Church* (New York: Harper & Row, 1970); Nigel Aston, *Religion and Revolution in France, 1780–1804* (Washington: Catholic University Press, 2000); Dale Van Kley, "Christianity as Casualty and Chrysalis of Modernity: The Problem of Dechristianization in the French Revolution," *American Historical Review* 108 (October 2003): 1081–1104.

54. For example, Noah Shusterman points to the October 10 decree as one of the first steps in the de-Christianization movement. *The French Revolution: Faith, Desire, and Politics* (New York: Routledge, 2014), 206.

55. Copies of Fouché's arrêté were printed in several newspapers, including the 18 October 1793 editions of *Journal de la montagne* and *Moniteur universel.* It has also been reprinted in many monographs, including Madeleine Lassère, *Villes et cimetières en France de l'Ancien Régime à nos jours* (Paris: Éditions l'Harmattan, 1997), 74.

56. In his classic text, François Alphonse Aulard surmised that Chaumette was probably the one who inspired Fouché's radical anti-Catholic activity. *Le culte de la raison et le culte de l'être suprême, 1793–1794: Essai historique* (Paris: F. Alcan, 1892), 26. For a more complicated analysis of the origins of de-Christianization, see Nicole Bossut, "Aux origines de la déchristianisation dans le Nièvre: Fouché, Chaumette, ou les jacobins nivernais?" *Annales historiques de la Révolution française* 264 (1986): 181–202.

57. "Commune de Paris. Conseil-général du 27 du premier mois," *Gazette nationale ou Le Moniteur universel* 30 (21 October 1793), reprinted in *Réimpression de l'ancien Moniteur,* vol. 18 (Paris: Bureau central, 1841), 161.

58. "Commune de Paris. Conseil-général du 1er frimaire," *Gazette nationale ou Le Moniteur universel* 63 (23 November 1793), reprinted in *Réimpression de l'ancien Moniteur,* vol. 18 (Paris: Bureau central, 1841), 482.

59. "Suite du Discours prononcé part Robespierre, à la convention nationale, dans la séance du 8 thermidor," *Journal des débats et des décrets* 724 (9 September 1794): 475.

60. Jean-Marie Coupé, *Des sépultures en politique et en morale* (Paris: Imprimerie nationale, 1796), 4.

61. Jean-Charles Laveaux, "Sur les sépultures des grands hommes, et celles des autres citoyens," *Journal de la montagne* 48 (19 July 1793).

62. John Shovlin, *The Political Economy of Virtue: Luxury, Patriotism, and the Origins of the French Revolution* (Ithaca, NY: Cornell University Press, 2006), 61.

63. John Iverson, "Introduction to the Forum on Emulation in France, 1750–1800," *Eighteenth-Century Studies* 36, no. 2 (2003): 220.

64. Nira Kaplan, "Virtuous Competition among Citizens: Emulation in Politics and Pedagogy during the French Revolution," *Eighteenth-Century Studies* 36, no. 2 (2003): 245–46. The seminal work on festivals remains Mona Ozouf, *Festivals and the French Revolution,* trans. Alan Sheridan (Cambridge, MA: Harvard University Press, 1988).

65. Jean-Baptiste Avril, *Rapport de l'administration des travaux publics, sur les cimetières; lu au Conseil-général par le citoyen Avril* (Paris, 1794).

66. Ibid., 6–7.

67. Lassère, *Villes et cimetières en France,* 78.

68. Avril, *Rapport sur les cimetières,* 11.

69. "Convention nationale. Présidence de Ruhl. Suite de la séance du 20 ventôse," *Gazette nationale ou Le Moniteur universel* 172 (12 March 1794), reprinted in *Réimpression de l'ancien Moniteur,* vol. 19 (Paris: Bureau central, 1841), 672.

70. AN F13 908, "Rapport présenté au ministre de l'Intérieur," 11 prairial, year IV (30 May 1796).

71. Jean-Jacques Coindre, *Mémoire sur la translation des cimetières hors de la ville de Lyon* (Lyon, 1789).

72. Willermoz, Dutreih, Roux, and Carret, *Les Commissaires aux inhumations, aux citoyens maire et officiers municipaux de Commune-Afranchie* (Lyon: Imprimerie républicaine, 1794), 16.

Chapter 2. The Solution of the Dead

1. Gaspard-Gilbert Delamalle, *Réflexions sur l'enterrement de ma mère: Ou, sur les cérémonies et la moralité des institutions civiles en générale,* 2nd ed. (Paris: Librairie Chrétienne, year 4 [1795–96]), 4–6. The first edition of this essay was published in 1794 and printed by Boulard.

2. Ibid., 9.

3. Joseph Clarke, *Commemorating the Dead in Revolutionary France, 1789–1799* (Cambridge: Cambridge University Press, 2007). Clarke argues that Revolutionary attempts to create an alternative to Catholic burial culture were a tragic failure. Thomas Kselman makes a similar argument, although Kselman also interprets the postrevolutionary period as the early stage of a broader "rechristianization of the cemetery" in France. "The Dechristianization of Death in Modern France," in *The Decline of Christianity in Modern Europe,* ed. Hugh McLeod (Cambridge: Cambridge University Press, 2004), 145–62.

4. Delamalle, *Réflexions sur l'enterrement de ma mère,* 8.

5. AN F13 330, "Pétition à la convention nationale sur les cimetières," 11 floréal, year 2 (30 April 1794).

6. For more on Picpus, see Ronen Steinberg, "Spaces of Mourning: The Cemetery of Picpus and the Memory of the Terror in Post-Revolutionary France," *Proceedings of the Western Society for French History* 36 (2008): 133–47.

7. Daniel Arasse, *The Guillotine and the Terror,* trans. Christopher Miller (London: Allen Lane, 1989), 108.

8. AN F13 330, Letter of 21 messidor, year II (9 July 1794).

9. AN F13 524, Letter from Riédain to "citoyens législateurs." Although this letter is undated, it was received by various concerned parties on 29 germinal (18 April) and 1 floréal (20 April) of year III (1795).

10. AN F13 524, Letter from the Architect Poyet to the Commission of Public Works, 7 vendémiaire, year IV (29 September 1795). The Ministry of the Interior quickly approved

Riédain's request for an indemnity but repeatedly denied his requests for an increase in funds to compensate for things such as his lost fruit trees.

11. Bronislaw Baczko, *Ending the Terror: The French Revolution after Robespierre*, trans. Michel Petheram (Cambridge: Cambridge University Press, 1994); Ronald Schechter, "Gothic Thermidor: The Bals des victimes, the Fantastic, and the Production of Historical Knowledge in Post-Terror France," *Representations* 61 (winter 1998): 78–94; Joseph Zizek, "'Plum de Fer': Louis-Marie Prudhomme Writes the French Revolution," *French Historical Studies* 24, no. 3 (2003): 619–60; Ronen Steinberg, "Reckoning with Terror: Retribution, Redress, and Remembrance in Post-Revolutionary France," in *Oxford Handbook of the French Revolution*, ed. David Andress (Oxford: Oxford University Press, 2015), 487–502; Lela Greybill, *The Visual Culture of Violence after the French Revolution* (New York: Routledge, 2016).

12. Charles-Joseph Trouvé, "Des honneurs que l'on doit render aux morts," *Gazette nationale ou Le Moniteur universel* 206 (16 April 1795), reprinted in *Réimpression de l'ancien Moniteur*, vol. 24 (Paris: Plon, 1856), 202.

13. Andrew Jainchill, *Reimagining Politics after the Terror: The Republican Origins of French Liberalism* (Ithaca, NY: Cornell University Press, 2008); Pierre Serna, *La République des girouettes (1789–1815 et au-delà), une anomalie politique: La France de l'extrême centre* (Paris: Champ Vallon, 2005); Howard G. Brown and Judith A. Miller, eds., *Taking Liberties: Problems of a New Order from the French Revolution to Napoleon* (Manchester: Manchester University Press, 2002); Isser Woloch, *The New Regime: Transformations in the French Civic Order, 1789–1820s* (New York: W. W. Norton, 1995).

14. AN F13 908, "Rapport présenté au ministre de l'intérieur" 11 prairial, year IV (30 May 1796).

15. AN F13 908, "Extrait de la séance du 4 fructidor, an IV, Administration municipale du canton de Clichy" (21 August 1796).

16. AN F13 908, "Administration municipale du 1er arrondissement, commissaire du directoire exécutif au citoyen ministre de l'intérieur" (undated, but year 4 [1795–96]).

17. AN F13 908. There are a series of letters between different branches of the municipal and national government discussing this issue. The above quotations come from an undated letter from the municipal administration of the first arrondissement to the minister of the interior. The cemetery near parc Monceau was eventually closed down in the spring of 1797. It was replaced by a new cemetery at the base of Montmartre that was the first incarnation of the still-existing Montmartre Cemetery.

18. Jacques-Michel Coupé, *Des sépultures en politique et en morale* (Paris: Imprimerie nationale, 1796), 2, 3, 10.

19. Emmanuel Pastoret, *Rapport sur la violation des sépultures et des tombeaux, fait aux nom de la commission de la classification et de la révision des lois* (Paris: Imprimerie nationale, 1796).

20. Jean-Baptiste LaFargue, *Motion d'ordre sur la police des cimetières et des inhumations* (Paris: Imprimerie nationale, 1798), 3–4.

21. Le C . . . [Marie-Nicolas-Silvestre Guillon], *Sur le respect dû aux tombeaux; et l'indécence des inhumations actuelles. Nouvelle édition, augmentée de la sépulture et de la mélancolie, poèmes de Legouvé* (Paris, year VIII [1799–1800]), 4.

22. Arsenne Thiébaut, *Réflexions sur les pompes funèbres* (Paris: Galetti, year VI [1797–98]), 4.

23. Gabriel-Marie Legouvé, "La sépulture," 4. Legouvé was an early member of the Institut de France (since 1798) and was most known for his poem exalting the virtues of women, "Le mérite des femmes" (1801). However, he also penned two elegiac poems dedicated to darker subjects: "La Sépulture" in 1798 and "La Mélancolie" in 1800. *Les souvenirs, la sépulture et la mélancolie* (Paris: Lemierre, year VI [1797–98]).

24. Jacques Cambry, *Rapport sur les sépultures: Présenté à l'administration centrale du département de la Seine* (Paris, year 7 [1798–99]), 1–2.

25. An otherwise comprehensive description of Napoleonic civil reforms is Isser Woloch's *The New Regime,* but Woloch's book contains virtually no information about cemetery or burial reform.

26. These pamphlets were previously analyzed by Pascal Hintermeyer, *Politiques de la mort: Tirées du concours de l'Institut, germinal an VIII–vendémiaire an IX* (Paris: Payot, 1981).

27. One of the most thorough analyses of the Moral and Political Sciences Class of the National Institute is Martin S. Staum, *Minerva's Message: Stabilizing the French Revolution* (Montreal: McGill-Queen's University Press, 1996).

28. For example, when Parisian entrepreneur Citizen Schèdre wrote to the minister of the interior in early 1800 requesting a meeting to discuss his plan for private tombs, the minister responded by suggesting that Schèdre submit his ideas to the institute for consideration. AN F1cl I87.

29. "Dictionnaires d'autrefois," The ARTFL Project, http://artfl-project.uchicago.edu/node/17.

30. Sarah Maza, *The Myth of the French Bourgeoisie: An Essay on the Social Imaginary* (Cambridge, MA: Harvard University Press, 2003), 59; Jainchill, *Reimagining Politics after the Terror,* 62–107.

31. AIF 1H5 b, Mollès, 2–3. The entries to the institute competition are all collected in the Archives de l'Institut de France under the call numbers 1H5, 1H6, and 1H7. Only the last name of each author is indicated.

32. Coupé, *Des sépultures en politique et en morale,* 5.

33. Coupé, *De la moralité des sépultures et de leur police* (Paris: C. Vollant, 1800), 22.

34. François-Valentin Mulot, *Vues d'un citoyen, ancien député de Paris à l'Assemblée legislative, sur les sépultures* (Paris: Imprimerie de la rue des Droits de l'homme, 1797), 20.

35. AIF 1H6 19, Doderet, 4.

36. Général Pommereul, *Mémoire sur les funérailles. Question proposée par le Ministère, et jugée par l'Institut, le 15 vendémiaire, an 9* (Tours: Billault jeune, year IX [1800–1801]), 11.

37. AIF 1H7 40, Pagès, 3.

38. AIF 1H7 37, Magouet-Magouerie, 9.

39. Review of Joseph Girard, *Des tombeaux,* L'Esprit des journaux français et étrangères par une société de gens de lettres 4 (January 1802): 39–45.

40. Joseph de Girard, *Des tombeaux: Ou, de l'influence des institutions funèbres sur les moeurs* (Paris: F. Buisson, 1801), 36–38.

41. Ibid., 38–39.

42. Ibid., 53–54.

43. Pierre-Louis Roederer, *Des institutions funéraires convenables a une république qui permet tous les cultes, et n'adopte aucun: mémoire lu par Roederer, dans la séance publique de l'Institut national des sciences et des arts, le 25 Messidor, l'an IV* (Paris, year IV [1796]).

44. Jacques-Olivier Boudon, *Napoléon et les cultes: Les religions en Europe à l'aube du XIXe siècle (1800–1815)* (Paris: Fayard, 2002).

45. Pierre Dolivier, *Essai sur les funérailles* (Versailles, year IX [1800–1801]). For more on Dolivier's activity during the Revolution, see David Hunt, "The People and Pierre Dolivier: Popular Uprisings in the Seine-et-Oise Department (1791–1792)," *French Historical Studies* 11, no. 2 (autumn 1979): 184–214; and Maurice Dommanget and Michel Vovelle, *Enragés et curés rouges en 1793: Jacques Roux, Pierre Dolivier* (Paris: Spartacus, 1993).

46. In his foreword (*avant propos*) Dolivier refers to "morales publiques," not "moeurs."

47. Dolivier, *Essai sur les funérailles,* 52–54.

48. Ibid., 66.

49. Staum, *Minerva's Message*, 68.

50. AIF 1H6 25, Le Citoyen X. . . . S. . . . S . . . , 7.

51. AIF 1H6 19, Doderet, 54.

52. Thomas Doderet, *Catéchisme de toutes les religions en abrégé, dédié au Cercle constitutionnel de la commune de Langres* (Chaumont: Imprimerie de Cousot, year VI [1797–98]).

53. AIF 1H6 19, Doderet, 20.

54. Dolivier, *Essai sur les funérailles*, 66.

55. AIF 1H6 19, Doderet, 24.

56. Ibid., 8.

57. Pommereul, *Mémoire sur les funérailles*, 32, 34.

58. In addition to the essays already mentioned, the notion of separate cemeteries also occurred in essays by Doulgelet from Le Mans, who suggested that the cemetery for the wicked be razed to the ground (AIF 1H6 20). Siozard (AIF 1H7 33), Bonnard (AIF 1H5 15), and Laurier (AIF 1H5 12) all proposed similar provisions for the separation of the good and wicked.

59. A.-J. Ronesse, *Projet pour les sépultures* (Paris: Debray, year IX [1800–1801]), 39.

60. AIF 1H6 18, Gaignoeux, 13.

61. AIF 1H6 23, Anonymous, 74.

62. In addition to the essays about emulation cited in chapter 1, see David A. Bell, *The Cult of the Nation in France: Inventing Nationalism, 1680–1800* (Cambridge, MA: Harvard University Press, 2003), 107–39.

63. Richard Etlin, *Symbolic Space: French Enlightenment Architecture and Its Legacy* (Chicago: University of Chicago Press, 1994).

64. Coupé, *De la moralité des sépultures*, 30.

65. François-Antoine Daubermesnil, *Corps législatif. Conseil des cinq-cents. Rapport sur les inhumations. Séance du 21 brumaire an V* (Paris: Imprimerie nationale, 1797), 11.

66. Ibid., 10.

67. Mulot, *Vues d'un citoyen sur les sépultures*, 4.

68. Girard, *Essai sur les sépultures*, 113.

69. Dolivier, *Essai sur les funérailles*, 1.

70. Ibid., 24–25.

71. Charles Bauchal, *Nouveau dictionnaire biographique et critique des architects français* (Paris: Librairie générale de l'architecture, 1887), 659.

72. Pierre Giraud, *Pétition du citoyen Giraud, ci-devant architecte du département de Paris, à la Convention nationale* (Paris: Veuve Hérissant, 1794), 7.

73. Pierre Giraud, *Essai sur les sépultures: Composé en l'an IV, et deposé au département de la Seine, le 11 nivôse, an VII, avec les plans, coupes, et élévations du monument projeté* (Paris: Paris: R. Jacquin, 1799); Pierre Giraud, *Les tombeaux, ou essai sur les sépultures. Ouvrage dans lequel l'auteur rappelle les coutumes des anciens peuples; cite sommairement celles observées par les modernes; donne les procédés pour dissoudre les chairs, calciner les ossements humains, les convertir en une substance indestructible, et en composer le médaillon de chaque individu*, 2nd ed. (Paris: Desenne, 1801).

74. Giraud, *Les tombeaux*, 21.

75. Giraud, *Essai sur les sépultures*, 9. This anecdote does not appear in the second, revised and expanded edition of Giraud's essay from 1801.

76. Giraud, *Les tombeaux*, 18–19.

77. Ibid., 20.

78. Cambry, *Rapport sur les sépultures*, 11.

79. AN F8 92, "Projet présenté au ministre de l'intérieur le 25 prairial, an VIII" (14 June 1800).

80. Richard A. Etlin, *The Architecture of Death: The Transformation of the Cemetery in Eighteenth-Century Paris* (Cambridge, MA: MIT Press, 1984), 273; Thomas A. Kselman, *Death and the Afterlife in Modern France* (Princeton, NJ: Princeton University Press, 1993).

81. F.-X. de Feller, Charles Weiss, and l'abbé Busson, *Biographie universelle, ou, dictionnaire historique des hommes qui se sont fait un nom par leur génie, leurs talents, leurs vertus, leurs erreurs ou leurs crimes*, vol. 3 (Paris: Gaume Frères, 1848), 659.

82. Edward A. Whitcombe, "Napoleon's Prefects," *American Historical Review* 79, no. 4 (October 1974): 1103.

83. Nicolas Frochot, *Arrêté du préfet du département de la Seine concernant les inhumations* (Paris: 21 ventôse, an IX [12 March 1801]), 1.

84. Ibid., 2.

85. Ibid., 3, 10. For more on the development of the private funeral business in early nineteenth-century France, see Kselman, *Death and the Afterlife in Modern France*, chapter 6, "The Origins of Commercial Funerals," 222–56.

86. Kselman, *Death and the Afterlife in Modern France*, 228.

87. Napoleon Bonaparte, "Décret impérial sur les sépultures," 23 prairial an XII, *Collection des lois, senatus-consultes, décrets impériaux et avis du conseil d'état relatifs aux cultes; publiés depuis le concordat jusqu'au 1er janvier 1813* (Paris: Rivals, 1813), 180–84.

88. *Rapport fait par les citoyens Hallé, Desessartz, Toulogeon, Reviellère-Lepaux, Leblond et Camus, commissaires chargés par l'Institut national des sciences et arts, de l'examen des mémoires envoyés au concours proposé par le gouvernement, sur les questions relatives aux cérémonies funéraires et aux lieux des sépultures. Jugement porté par l'Institut et proclamation du prix* (Paris: Bailleul, 1800), 4.

Chapter 3. The City of the Dead

1. M*****, *Le cimetière de la Madeleine* (Paris, 1800), 125. The Madeleine Cemetery is most famous for being the burial site of Louis XVI and Marie Antoinette, although it also contained the bodies of the Girondins and others executed while the guillotine was located at Place de la Révolution (present-day place de la Concorde). Since this particular cemetery is usually associated with the Royalist reaction, M***'s conciliatory tone is particularly noteworthy.

2. J. G. Warin, *Le cimetière de la Madeleine* (Paris: Le Petit Jeune, 1800).

3. For more on the reactionary and revenge-fueled violence of the 1790s, see Bronislaw Baczko, *Ending the Terror: The French Revolution after Robespierre*, trans. Michael Petheram (Cambridge: Cambridge University Press, 1994); Howard G. Brown, *Ending the French Revolution: Violence, Justice, and Repression from the Terror to Napoleon* (Charlottesville: University of Virginia Press, 2006); Ronen Steinberg, "Reckoning with Terror: Retribution, Redress, and Remembrance in Post-Revolutionary France," in *Oxford Handbook of the French Revolution*, ed. David Andress (Oxford: Oxford University Press, 2015), 487–502.

4. M*****, *Le cimetière de la Madeleine*, 71.

5. For an analysis of why *union et oubli* failed, see David Skuy, *Assassination, Politics, and Miracles: France and the Royalist Reaction of 1820* (Montreal: McGill-Queen's University Press, 2003); and Sheryl Kroen, *Politics and Theatre: The Crisis of Legitimacy in Restoration France, 1815–1830* (Berkeley: University of California Press, 2000). Another influential work on the politics of the Restoration is Pierre Rosanvallon's *La monarchie impossible: Les chartes de 1814 et de 1830* (Paris: Fayard, 1994).

6. In addition to the books about death, commemoration, and cemeteries in nineteenth-century France, a brief reading list of dominant works about the history of Père Lachaise and the "cemetery cult" include Vincent LaGlande, *Histoire du Père Lachaise* (Paris: Vermet, 1988); Danielle Tartakowsky, *Nous irons chanter sur vos tombes: Le Père Lachaise XIXe–XXe siècle* (Paris: Le grand livre du mois, 2000). An excellent edited collection covering the entire history of the cemetery and associated themes is Katherine Healey, Karen Bowie, and Agnès Bos, eds., *Le Père Lachaise* (Paris: Action artistique de la ville de Paris, 1998).

7. M. P. St.-A. [Pierre-François Piétresson de Saint-Aubin], *Promenade aux cimetières de Paris, aux sépultures royales de Saint-Denis, et aux Catacombes* (Paris: Panckoucke, 1816), 27–31. Descriptions of Eliza Veroquier's tomb appear in other early nineteenth-century descriptions of Parisian cemeteries, including an 1817 publication that also makes note of the penciled-in epitaph: C. P. Arnaud, *Recueil de tombeaux des quatre cimetières de Paris, avec leurs épitaphes et leurs inscriptions*, vol. 1 (Paris: Arnaud, 1817), 74. Arnaud also describes the impromptu epitaph that M. P. de St.-A. claims to have inscribed on Eliza's tomb. He notes that the penciled-in epitaph was dated December 1811, which is why I indicated that M. P. de St.-A.'s visit took place in 1811, despite publishing his account in 1825.

8. G.G., *Promenade sérieuse au cimetière du Père La Chaise, ou de Mont-Louis, près de Paris* (Paris: Imprimerie de Lachevardière fils, 1826), 22.

9. François-Marie Marchant de Beaumont, *Vues pittoresques, historiques, et morales du cimetière du P. La Chaise desinée par MM. Vigneront et Duplat, et gravées a l'aqua-tinta par M. Jazet et les meilleurs artistes* (Paris, 1821), 2.

10. Michel Ragon, *The Space of Death: A Study in Funerary Architecture, Decoration, and Urbanism*, trans. Alan Sheridan (Charlottesville: University Press of Virginia, 1983), 19.

11. For more on the strain to friendship in the postrevolutionary era, see Sarah Horowitz, *Friendship and Politics in Post-Revolutionary France* (University Park: Penn State University Press, 2013).

12. Régis Bertrand, "L'invention du cimetière français contemporain au Père-Lachaise au début du XIXe siècle," *Annales de l'Est* 2 (2012), 185.

13. On guidebooks in the postrevolutionary city, see Priscilla Ferguson, *Paris as Revolution: Writing the Nineteenth-Century City* (Berkeley: University of California Press, 1994), especially chapter 2, "Mapping the City," 36–79. Christopher Prendergrast also makes use of this source in *Paris and the Nineteenth Century* (Cambridge: Wiley-Blackwell, 1992).

14. For example, in *Death and the Afterlife in Modern France*, Thomas Kselman notes that it would be "misleading" to rely on epitaphs and tombs to "tell us about the sentiments that people of the past had toward their dead" (165).

15. Antoine Caillot, *Voyage religieux et sentimentale aux quatre cimetières de Paris* (Paris, 1809), 225.

16. Ibid., 337, 340.

17. Ibid., 14.

18. Ibid., 99, 68, 157.

19. Ibid., 188.

20. Antoine Caillot, *Mémoire pour servir à l'histoire des moeurs et usages français*, vol. 1 (Paris: Dauvin, 1827), 50–53.

21. Rebecca Spang, "The Frivolous French: 'Liberty of Pleasure' and the End of Luxury," in *Taking Liberties: Problems of a New Order from the French Revolution to Napoleon*, ed. Howard G. Brown and Judith A. Miller (Manchester: Manchester University Press, 2002), 111.

22. Ibid., 122.

23. Caillot, *Voyage religieux et sentimentale*, 37–38.

24. Ibid., 43–52.

25. Ibid., 109, 85.

26. Ibid., "Avertissement."

27. "Variétés, revue du mois," *Mercure de France* 34 (1808), 276.

28. Caillot, *Voyage religieux et sentimentale*, 160.

29. For Parisian tombstones during the Old Regime, an invaluable resource is *Épitaphier du vieux Paris: Recueil général des inscriptions funéraires des églises, couvents, collèges, hospices, cimetières et charniers, depuis le moyen âge jusqu'à la fin du XVIIIe siècle*, ed. Emile Raunier, 3 vols. (Paris, 1890–1901). For an analysis of this source, see Agnès Verlet, *Pierres parlantes: Florilège d'épitaphes parisiennes du Moyen Age à la fin du XVIIIe siècle* (Paris: Commission des travaux historiques, 2000).

30. F.-G.-T. de Jolimont, *Les mausolées français: Recueil des tombeaux les plus remarquables par leur structure, leurs épitaphes ou les cendres qu'ils contiennent, érigés dans les nouveaux cimetières de Paris* (Paris: Firmin-Didot, 1821). There are no page numbers in this book.

31. For more on family and friendship as a source of solidarity, see Horowitz, *Friendship and Politics*; Suzanne Desan, *The Family on Trial in Revolutionary France* (Berkeley: University of California Press, 2006); Pierre Rosanvallon, *The Demands of Liberty: Civil Society in France since the Revolution*, trans. Arthur Goldhammer (Cambridge, MA: Harvard University Press, 2007).

32. M. M. Roger, père et fils, *Le Champ du repos, ou le cimetière Mont-Louis dit du Père Lachaise, ouvrage orné avec de planches, représentant plus de 2000 mausolées érigés dans ce cimetière, depuis sa création jusqu'au 1er janvier, 1816, avec leurs épitaphes; son plan topographique, tel qu'il existait du temps du père delachaise, et tel qu'il existe aujourd'hui; précédé du portrait de ce jésuite, d'un abrégé de sa vie; et suivi de quelques remarques sur la manière dont différens peuples honorent les défunts*, vol. 2 (Paris: Pillet, 1816), 121.

33. Ibid., 25.

34. Ibid., 370.

35. Jacques-Antoine Dulaure, *Histoire physique, civile, et morale de Paris: depuis les premiers temps, tome quatrième* (Brussels: Baudouin, 1825), 234–36.

36. Marchant de Beaumont, *Vues pittoresques*, 136.

37. Roger, *Le Champ de repos*, vol. 1, epigram.

38. AP VD 4 10 no. 2876. *Arrête* of 15 ventôse, year 13 (6 March 1805).

39. For example, in an 1806 decree on church services for the dead, indigents were repeatedly guaranteed a free and decent funeral and burial. *Ministère des cultes, Extrait des minutes de la secrétairerie d'état au palais de Saint-Cloud, le 18 mai 1806*. AN F19 4379.

40. *Recherches statistiques sur la ville de Paris et le département de la Seine* (Paris: Imprimerie royale, 1826), tableau 61.

41. Maxime du Camp, *Paris, ses organes, ses fonctions, et sa vie dans la seconde moitié du XIXe siècle, t. VI* (Paris: Hachette, 1875), 140.

42. Marchant de Beaumont, *Vues pittoresques*, 103–4.

43. Roger, *Le champ de repos*, vol. 2, 61–62.

44. Arnaud, *Recueil de tombeaux*, vol. 1, 18.

45. Roger, *Le champ de repos*, vol. 2, 14.

46. Arnaud, *Recueil de tombeaux*, vol. 1, 50–51.

47. Roger, *Le champ de repos*, vol. 2, 8.

48. Ibid., 15.

49. Roger, *Le champ de repos*, vol. 1, 116.

50. Ibid., 245.

51. Ibid., vol. 2, 323.

52. Ibid., 361.

53. Ibid., vol. 1, 275. Lagrange's tomb is still standing in Père Lachaise. It can be found in the twenty-ninth division of the cemetery.

54. Arnaud, *Recueil de tombeaux,* vol. 1, 34–36.

55. Ibid., 34.

56. Marchant de Beaumont, *Vues pittoresques,* 338.

57. Roger, *Le champ de repos,* vol. 2, 47.

58. On sentimentalism, see Anne Vincent-Buffault, *A History of Tears: Sensibility and Sentimentality in France* (Hampshire: Macmillan, 1991); David Denby, *Sentimental Narrative and the Social Order in France, 1760–1820* (Cambridge: Cambridge University Press, 1994); and William Reddy, *The Invisible Code: Honor and Sentiment in Postrevolutionary France, 1814–1848* (Berkeley: University of California Press, 1994).

59. Piétresson de Saint-Aubin, *Promenade aux cimetières de Paris,* "Avertissement."

60. Arnaud, *Recueil de tombeaux,* vol. 2, 87–88, 96, 94.

61. Roger, *Le champ de repos,* vol. 2, 285, 300.

62. Piétresson de Saint-Aubin, *Promenade aux cimetières de Paris,* 101.

63. Arnaud, *Recueil de tombeaux,* vol. 1, preface.

64. François-Marie Marchant de Beaumont, *Le conducteur au cimetière de l'est, ou du Père Lachaise* (Paris: Plassan, 1820), 75–77.

65. Marchant de Beaumont, *Vues pittoresques,* 353.

66. Ibid., 344–48.

67. Marchant de Beaumont, *Le conducteur au cimetière de l'est,* 35.

68. Caillot, *Voyage religieux et sentimentale,* 93.

69. Marchant de Beaumont, *Le conducteur au cimetière de l'est,* 425–26.

70. Rogers, *Le Champ de repos,* vol. 1, iii.

71. Alexandre-Théodore Brogniart, *Plans du palais de la Bourse de Paris, et du cimetière Mont-Louis en six planches* (Paris: Crapelet, 1814), 8.

72. Dr. H. Bayard, "Memoire sur la police des cimetières," *Annales d'hygiène publique et de médecine légale,* vol. 17 (Paris: J.-B. Baillière, 1837), 299, 301.

Chapter 4. The Empire of the Dead

1. Etienne de Jouy, "Les Catacombes," in *L'Hermite de la Chaussée-d'Antin, ou, Observations sur les moeurs et les usages parisiennes au commencement du XIXe siècle,* vol. 2 (Paris: Pilet, 1814), 361.

2. François-marie Marchant [de Beaumont], *Le conducteur de l'étranger à Paris* (Paris, 1815), 249–51.

3. Louis-Étienne Héricart de Thury, "Précis historique sur les Catacombes de Paris," in *Catacombes de Paris, registre de visiteurs, 1809–1813,* BHVP MSS 11, 51, 80, 76. The Catacombs Registry, which can be found in the archives of the Bibliothèque Historique de la Ville de Paris, is handwritten with the front of each page numbered by hand. It will henceforth be referred to as *Registre* in the footnotes.

4. "Album," *Revue des deux mondes, journal des voyages, des sciences, de l'administration, des moeurs, etc . . . chez les différents peuples du globe, par une société de savants* 2, no. 2 (1830), 424.

5. John Griscom, *A Year in Europe: Comparing a Journal of Observations in England, Scotland, Ireland, France, Switzerland, and the North of Italy, and Holland. In 1818 and 1819* (New York: Collins, 1823), 66.

6. *Mémoires historiques de l'abbé Artigny*, quoted in Émile Gérards, *Les Catacombes de Paris* (Paris: Chamuel, 1892), 37–38.

7. AN F13 742 "Ordonnance concernant les carrières du 2 ventôse, an IX."

8. Jacques-Antoine Dulaure, *Histoire civile, physique et morale de Paris, depuis les premiers temps jusqu'à nos jours*, 2nd ed., vol. 9 (Paris: Guillaume, 1824), 218; *Histoire de Paris et de ses monuments, nouvelle édition refondue et complété jusqu'à nos jours par L. Batissier* (Paris: Furne, 1846), 603.

9. Marc Viré, preface to *Description des Catacombes de Paris précédée d'un précis historique sur les catacombes de tous les peuples de l'ancien et du nouveau continent*, by Héricart de Thury (Paris, 1815; reprint with preface, Paris: CTHS, 2005), 9.

10. AN F13 742 "Rapport présenté au Ministre de l'Intérieur." The various reports that refer to this Menilmontant incident all reference Guillaumot's printed report, 46.

11. AN F13 203 L. C. F. Héricart de Thury, "Rapport sur les travaux des carrières de Paris et environs," 1810.

12. Viré, "Préface."

13. Villedieu, *Projet de catacombes pour la ville de Paris en adaptant à cet usage les carrières qui se trouvent tant dans son enceinte que dans ses environs* (Paris, 1782), 6.

14. "Thury on the Catacombs of Paris," *English Review and London Critical Journal* 7, no. 13 (1816): 131.

15. AN F13 742, "Rapport fait au Conseil des bâtiments civils, sur l'état actuel des carrières qui se trouvent sous Paris, 26 frimaire, an VI."

16. AN F13 742, "Rapport au Directoire exécutive, par le ministre de l'Intérieur."

17. AN F13 742, "Rapport présenté au ministre de l'Intérieur, 25 ventôse, an VI."

18. AN F13 742, "Préfet de police au ministre de l'Intérieur, 22 nivôse, an X."

19. *Registre*, 3.

20. Most descriptions of the Catacombs contain similar timelines about the order in which bones made their way into the Catacombs. The most comprehensive of these is Gérards, *Les Catacombes de Paris*, 139–61. Gérards's book contains information up to 1878. Thury's *Description des Catacombes* contains information up to 1813.

21. Héricart de Thury, *Description des Catacombes de Paris*, xvi.

22. Gilles Thomas and Xavier Ramette, "La Création et l'aménagement des Catacombes. Premier musée souterrain de France au début de l'Empire, sous l'égide de L.É.F. Héricart Ferrand, entre 1809 et 1815," *Napoleonica. La Revue* 10 (2011): 75.

23. "Thury on the Catacombs of Paris," 142.

24. de Jouy, "Les Catacombes," 364.

25. T.H. "Fragments Illustrative of Paris, in 1814: The Catacombs," *New Monthly Magazine and Universal Register* 22 (1815): 311.

26. AN F14 2728 1, letter of April 10, 1818.

27. Aimé Guillon, *Les Martyrs de la foi pendant la Révolution française, ou, Martyrologie des pontifs, prêtres, religieux, religieuses, laïcs de l'un et l'autre sexe, qui périrent alors pour la foi* (Paris: G. Mathiot, 1821), 185.

28. *Registre*, 4, 89, 90.

29. Ibid., 118, 119.

30. Seth Williams Stevenson, *Journal of a Tour Through Part of France, Flanders, and Holland, Including a Visit to Paris, and a Walk over the Field of Waterloo: Made in the Summer of 1816* (Norwich: Norfolk Chronicle Press, 1817), 175.

31. *Registre*, 26v.

32. The best-known nineteenth-century fictionalizations of the Catacombs are Elie Berthet, *Les Catacombes de Paris* (Paris, 1854); Joseph Méry, *Salons et souterrains de Paris*

(Paris: Schiller, 1851); Alexandre Dumas, *Les Mohicans de Paris* (Paris: Michel Lévy frères, 1871); and Pierre Zaccone, *Les drames des catacombes* (Paris: Balay aîné, 1863).

33. *Catacombs*, directed by Tomm Coker and David Elliot (Lion's Gate Film, 2007); Jack Manini and Michel Chevereau, *Catacombes Tome 1: Le diable vert* (Paris: Glénat, 2010), and Jack Manini, *Catacombes Tome 2* (Paris: Glénat, 2011); Neal Shea, "Under Paris," *National Geographic Magazine*, February 2011, 104–25; Natasha Gellig, "Paris Catacombs," smithsonian.com, March 28, 2014, http://www.smithsonianmag.com/travel/paris-catacombs-180950160/?no-ist.

34. *Registre*, 62v, 45v.

35. Jacques-Antoine Dulaure, *Panorama de la ville de Paris et guide de l'étranger à Paris* (Paris: P.-Corneille, 1824), 414.

36. *Registre*, 9.

37. M.P. de St.-A. [Pierre-François Piétresson de Saint-Aubin], *Promenade aux cimetières de Paris, aux sépultures royales de Saint-Denis et aux Catacombes* (Paris: Panckoucke, 1816), 233.

38. Ph. Chasles, "Les Catacombes de Saint-Michan," *Revue de Paris*, 2nd ed., vol. 3 (Paris: Levavasseur, 1830), 182.

39. Maurice Samuels, *The Spectacular Past: Popular History and the Novel in Nineteenth-Century France* (Ithaca, NY: Cornell University Press, 2004), 19–26; Vanessa Schwartz, *Spectacular Realities: Early Mass Culture in Fin-de-Siècle Paris* (Berkeley: University of California Press, 1998); Pamela Pilbeam, *Madame Tussaud and the History of the Waxworks* (London: Hambledon & London, 2003).

40. Samuels, *The Spectacular Past*, 26–27.

41. D. A. F. Sade, *Idées sur les romans*, ed. Octave Uzanne (Paris: Edouard Rouveyre, 1878), 32–33.

42. Griscom, *A Year in Europe*, 68.

43. Nestor Lamarque, "Les Catacombes de Paris," in *Paris, ou le livre des cent et un*, vol. 6 (Paris: Ladvocat, 1832), 20.

44. *Registre*, 85.

45. Piétresson de Saint-Aubin, *Promenade aux cimetières de Paris*, 222.

46. Peter Brooks, *The Melodramatic Imagination: Balzac, Henry James, Melodrama, and the Mode of Excess* (New Haven, CT: Yale University Press, 1995), 20.

47. *Memorandums of a Residence in France, in the Winter of 1815–1816, Including Remarks on French Manners and Society, with a Description of the Catacombs, and Notices of Some Other Objects of Curiosity and Works of Art, not Hitherto Described* (London: Longman, Hurst, Rees, Orme, and Brown, 1816), 320.

48. Félix Nadar, "Le Dessus et le dessous de Paris," in *Paris-Guide, par les principaux écrivains et artistes de la France*, vol. 2, *La vie* (Paris: A. Lacroix, 1867), 1572.

49. Thomas Détruisard, *Essai sur les Catacombes de Paris* (Paris, 1812), 17–18.

50. *Registre*, 79, 13v, 54v, 15v, 32v, 69.

51. Léon Thiessé, *Les Catacombes de Paris, poème en un chant* (Paris: Hocquet, 1815), 18.

52. M. Colnet [Charles Joseph Colnet du Ravel], "Le Cimetière des Innocents et les catacombes de Paris," in *L'Hermite du faubourg Saint-Germain, ou observations sur les moeurs et les usages français au commencement du XIXe siècle* (Paris: Pillet aîné, 1825), 226.

53. English translation from Henry Wadsworth Longfellow, *The Complete Poetical Works of Henry Wadsworth Longfellow, Cambridge Edition* (Boston, 1920), 629.

54. *Registre*, 29v, 43, 56v.

55. Jacques-Olivier Boudon, *Napoléon et les cultes: Les religions en Europe à l'aube du XIXe siècle (1800–1815)* (Paris: Fayard, 2002).

56. Héricart de Thury, *Description des Catacombes*, 223. A recent analysis of the inscriptions maintains that this unique "anthology" of funereal writings is as remarkable for its diversity as for its subterranean location. Ramette and Thomas, *Inscriptions des Catacombes de Paris: Arrête! C'est ici l'empire de la mort* (Paris: Cherche Midi, 2012), 23.

57. *Memorandums of a Residence in France*, 358; Stevenson, *Journal of a Tour through Part of France*, 174–75.

58. de Jouy, "Les Catacombes," 364; John Scott, *A Visit to Paris in 1814: Being a Review of the Moral, Political, Intellectual, and Social Condition of the French Capital* (Philadelphia: Edward Parker, 1815), lxvii.

59. *Registre*, 41.

60. Ibid., 41v, 54v, 104v, 108v, 132.

61. Ibid., 65.

62. Ibid., 41, 46, 55v, 123v.

63. Ibid., 20v.

64. Suzanne Glover Lindsay, *Funerary Arts and Tomb Cult: Living with the Dead in France, 1750–1870* (Burlington, VT: Ashgate, 2012), 24.

65. Jennifer Heuer, *The Family and the Nation: Gender and Citizenship in Revolutionary France* (Ithaca, NY: Cornell University Press, 2005); Suzanne Desan, *The Family on Trial in Revolutionary France* (Berkeley: University of California Press, 2006); Denise Davidson, *France after Revolution: Urban Life, Gender, and the New Social Order* (Cambridge, MA: Harvard University Press, 2007); June K. Burton, *Napoleon and the Woman Question: Discourses of the Other Sex in French Education, Medicine, and Medical Law, 1799–1815* (Lubbock: Texas Tech University Press, 2007).

66. Isser Woloch, *The New Regime: Transformations in the French Civic Order, 1789–1820s* (New York: W. W. Norton, 1994); James Livesey, *Making Democracy in the French Revolution* (Cambridge, MA: Harvard University Press, 2012); Robert Alexander, *Re-writing the French Revolution Tradition: Liberal Opposition and the Fall of the Bourbon Monarchy* (Cambridge: Cambridge University Press, 2004); Andrew Jainchill, *Reimagining Politics after the Terror* (Ithaca, NY: Cornell University Press, 2008).

67. Michel Foucault, *The Order of Things: An Archaeology of the Human Sciences* (New York: Vintage, 1970); Peter Fritzsche, *Stranded in the Present: Modern Time and the Melancholy of History* (Cambridge, MA: Harvard University Press, 2004).

68. Stephen Bann, *Romanticism and the Rise of History* (New York: Twayne, 1995).

69. "Le jour des morts dans les Catacombes de Paris," *Mercure de France* 58 (January 29, 1814), 193.

70. Thomas and Ramette, "Le creation et l'aménagement des catacombs," 51–52.

71. *Registre*, 53.

72. Héricart de Thury, *Description des Catacombes*, 280.

73. As David Lawrence Pike has noted, men of science like Cuvier and Buffon had recently begun to interpret the subterranean content of Paris as something constitutive of "history and meaning rather than merely pecuniary gain." "Paris Souterrain: Before and After the Revolution," *Dix-Neuf* 15, no. 2 (2011): 183.

74. *Registre*, 53v.

75. Ibid., 72v.

76. Ibid., 4v.

77. Détruisard, *Essai sur les Catacombes de Paris*, 7–8. A similar comment exists in Nestor de Lamarque, *Trois élégies* (Paris: Les librairies du Palais-royal, 1824), 7.

78. M. Gouriet, "Fragmens d'un voyage aux Catacombes de Paris," *Mercure de France* 67 (1816), 5. The *Mercure de France* indicates that this is an excerpt of a much longer piece in

prose and poetry that could be purchased at the author's house; however, no record of this publication appears in the BNF's catalog.

79. *Registre*, 83v.

80. Ibid., 79.

81. Ibid., 20v.

82. Ibid., 75.

83. Marchant de Beaumont, *Le Conducteur de l'étranger à Paris*, 249.

84. *Registre*, 96. Dominique Poulot has produced a comprehensive body of work on the development of *patrimoine* in France around the turn of the nineteenth century. In particular, see *Musée, nation, patrimoine (1789–1815)* (Paris: Gallimard, 1997), and *Une histoire du patrimoine en Occident, XVIIIe-XXIe siècle. Du monument aux valeurs* (Paris: Presses Universitaires de France, 2006). For work in English, see "The Birth of Heritage: 'le moment Guizot.' *Oxford Art Journal* 11, no. 2 (1998): 40–56.

85. *Registre*, 12.

86. Ibid., 82.

87. Ibid., 123.

88. Fabien Pillet, "Vers faits dans les Catacombes de Paris," *Almanach des muses pour 1819* 55 (1819): 208.

89. *Registre*, 22.

90. Ibid., 120v, 22.

91. Thomas and Ramette, "La Creation et l'aménagement des Catacombes," 120. Thomas and Ramette note that it was long believed that transfers to the Catacombs had stopped in 1859, but a photograph from 1957 shows a placard (now disappeared) indicating that bones were transferred from the "Cemetery of the East" (Père Lachaise Cemetery) as late as December 1933.

92. *Registre*, 90, 131.

93. Vanessa Harding, *The Dead and the Living in Paris and London, 1500–1670* (Cambridge: Cambridge University Press, 2002), 280, 105.

94. Eveline G. Bouwers, *Public Pantheons in Revolutionary Europe: Comparing Cultures of Remembrance, c. 1790–1840* (New York: Palgrave Macmillan, 2012), 5. Joseph Clarke makes a similar argument about the early years of the Panthéon in *Commemorating the Dead in Revolutionary France: Revolution and Remembrance, 1789–1799* (Cambridge: Cambridge University Press, 2007).

Chapter 5. The Museum of the Dead

1. Henry Redhead Yorke, *Letters from France, in 1802* (London: H. D. Symonds, 1804), 115.

2. Edmund John Eyre, *Observations Made at Paris during the Peace* (London: W. Meyler, 1803), 187.

3. Helena Maria Williams, *Sketches of the State of Manners and Opinions in the French Republic, towards the Close of the Eighteenth Century* (London: G. G. and J. Robinson, 1801), 235.

4. Notable works that investigate the place of the museum in the history of museums and art preservation include Andrew McClellan, *Inventing the Louvre: Art, Politics, and the Origins of the Modern Museum in Eighteenth-Century Paris* (Cambridge: Cambridge University Press, 1994); Francis Haskell, *History and Its Images: Art and the Interpretation of the Past* (New Haven, CT: Yale University Press, 1993); Stephen Bann, "Poetics of the Museum: Lenoir and Du Sommerard," *The Clothing of Clio: A Study of the Representation*

of History in Nineteenth-Century Britain and France (Cambridge: Cambridge University Press, 1984), 77–92.

5. Alexandra Stara, *The Museum of French Monuments, 1795–1816: Killing Art to Make History* (London: Routledge, 2013).

6. Louis-Sébastien Mercier, "Sur le dépôt des Petits-Augustins, dit: le Musée des Monuments Français," *Journal d'économie publique, de morale, et de politique*, vol. 5 (Paris: Journal de Paris, 1797), 327.

7. "Extraits des procès verbaux de l'assemblé législative de la convention nationale du 16 Septembre 1792," AN F17* 24 3.

8. "Rapport d'Alexandre Lenoir au Comité de l'instruction publique tendant à la création du Musée des Monuments français au Dépôt des Petits-Augustins" (1795), *Inventaire général des richesses d'art de la France: Archives du musée des monuments français*, vol. 1 (Paris: Plon, 1883), 24.

9. M. Bernier, "Municipalité de Paris. Administration des biens-nationaux ecclésiastiques. Bureau de liquidation. Extrait des délibérations du 25 et 26 juillet, 1791," AN F17* 24 3.

10. There is some disagreement about whether or not Lenoir was a Revolutionary. At the 1979 Consortium on Revolutionary Europe, Stanley Mellon delivered a paper on "Alexandre Lenoir versus the Revolution" and argued that despite its revolutionary origins, the Museum of French Monuments was essentially the antithesis of the revolution, dedicated to conservation rather than destruction. Commenting on Mellon's paper, Emmet Kennedy accurately pointed out that Lenoir had an ongoing and stable relationship with the central government, and that "Lenoir was not alone. He had a bureaucracy of conservation behind him, even during the Terror." Stanley Mellon, "Alexandre Lenoir: The Museum versus the Revolution," *The Consortium on Revolutionary Europe, 1750–1850*, vol. 9 (1979): 75–91.

11. AN F17* 24 4 no. 75, 6 January 1798, Letter to Alexandre Lenoir.

12. Henry Redhead Yorke, *Letters from France*, 111.

13. Henri Grégoire, *Rapport sur les destructions opérées par le Vandalisme, et sur les moyens de le réprimer* (Paris: Imprimerie nationale, 1794). For more on Grégoire and the invention of "vandalism" as a concept, see Anthony Vidler, "The Paradoxes of Vandalism: Henri Grégoire and the Thermidorian Discourse on Historical Monuments," in *The Abbé Grégoire and His World*, ed. Jeremy Popkin and Richard Popkin (Dordrecht: Kluwer, 2000), 129–56.

14. Alexandre Lenoir, "Rapport d'Alexandre Lenoir au comité de l'instruction publique tendant à la création du Musée des monuments français au dépôt des Petits-Augustins" (30 messidor, year III [18 July 1795]), in *Archives du Musée des monuments français*, vol. 1, 25.

15. Alexandre Lenoir, *Notice succincte des objets de sculpture et architecture réunis au dépôt provisoire national, rue des Petits-Augustins* (Paris: Desenne, 1793), 15.

16. Lenoir describes this event in a footnote of his 1810 catalog: *Musée impérial des monuments français: histoire des arts en France, et description chronologique des statues en marbre et en bronze, bas-reliefs et tombeaux des hommes et des femmes célèbres, qui sont réunis dans ce musée* (Paris: chez l'auteur, 1810), 252. Richelieu's head was then rumored to have been spirited away by a sympathetic citizen, who passed it on to a friend a year later. In 1866 the mummified head was presented to Napoleon III by the mayor of a small Breton village. It was finally returned to its original tomb in the Sorbonne in December 1866. Edmond Bonnaffé, "Les restes d'un grand homme," *Gazette des beaux-arts* 27 (April 1883): 324–26.

17. Jesse Goldhammer comments on the "neutralizing" violence committed against the royal corpses in *The Headless Republic* (Ithaca, NY: Cornell University Press 2005), 30.

18. Letter from Alexandre Lenoir, 30 frimaire, year II [20 December 1793], in *Archives du Musée des monuments français,* vol. 1, 17.

19. Ibid., 16. Two years later, Lenoir made a similar comment in a report to the Committee of Public Instruction, in which he requested funds to repair Francis I's tomb. "Please believe me, citizens, that it is not for the memory of Francis I that I ask to rebuild this monument which I will maintain for you; I forget his moeurs along with his remains." "Rapport d'Alexandre Lenoir au Comité de l'instruction publique tendant à la création du Musée des Monuments français au Dépôt des Petits-Augustins," in *Archives du Musée des monuments français*, vol. 1, 26.

20. AN F17 1280a, "Rapport sur le catalogue des Petits-Augustins, présenté par le citoyen Lenoir," 30 thermidor, year II [17 August 1794].

21. Mercier, "Sur le dépôt des Petits-Augustins," 327–28.

22. René de Chateaubriand, *Mémoires d'outre-tomb*, vol. 1 (Paris: Dufour, Mulat, et Boulanger, 1860), 314.

23. Alexandre Lenoir, *Notice historique des monuments des arts réunis au dépot national; rue des Petits-Augustins* (Paris: Desenne, year IV [1795]), vii–viii.

24. The whole affair of the Diane de Poitiers tomb is described, with documents, in *Archives du Musée des monuments français*, vol. 1, 86–93.

25. Another good example of this occurred in the summer of 1799 when someone sent a letter to Lenoir explaining how the tomb and remains of a famous poet, Fanteuil de Saint Victoire, had been sitting in a Jesuit abbey since their rescue during the Revolution. The citizen urged Lenoir to re-rescue this precious monument because it was being neglected in the abbey, whose occupants were using the tomb as a desk. AN F17*24 5, no. 100, Letter to Lenoir (29 fructidor, year VIII [16 September 1800]).

26. "Le préfet du département de la Seine-Inférieure au citoyen Lenoir, administrateur du Musée des Monuments français," 3 fructidor, year IX [21 August 1801], in *Archives du Musée des monuments français*, vol. 3, 17.

27. "Copie de la lettre écrite par le préfet de la Seine-Inférieure le 3 fructidor an IX, au Ministre de l'Intérieur" (21 August 1801), in *Archives du Musée des monuments français*, vol. 3, 18–20.

28. Ibid.

29. Haskell, *History and Its Images*, 246; Mellon, "Alexandre Lenoir," 82.

30. Antoine Quatremère de Quincy, *Rapport fait au conseil-général; le 15 thermidor, an 8, sur l'instruction publique, le rétablissement des bourses, le scandale des inhumations actuelles, l'érection de cimetières, la restitution des tombeaux, mausolées, etc.* (Paris: R. Jacquin, an VIII [1799–80]). Quatremère de Quincy puts forward a similar argument urging Napoleon not to strip Egypt and Italy of their arts in *Considérations morales sur la destination des ouvrages de l'art* (Paris: Crapelet, 1815).

31. Quatremère de Quincy, *Considerations morales*, 47–48; translation from Didier Maleuvre, *Museum Memories: History, Technology, Art* (Stanford, CA: Stanford University Press, 1999), 17.

32. René de Chateaubriand, *The Genius of Christianity*, trans. Charles White (Baltimore: John Murphy, 1856), 521.

33. Alexandre Lenoir, *Musée des monumens français, ou Description historique et chronologique des statues en marbre et en bronze, bas-reliefs et tombeaux des hommes et des femmes célèbres, pour server à l'histoire de France et à celle de l'art; ornée de gravures et augmentée d'une dissertation sur les costumes de chaque siècle* [henceforth MMF], vol. 2 (Paris: Guilleminet, 1801), 83. He also constructed a monument to Jean Goujon out of pieces of the sixteenth-century sculptor's own work and a bust that Lenoir had made in the early nineteenth century. Lenoir, *MMF*, vol. 3 (1802), 98–99.

34. Quatremère de Quincy, *Rapport fait au conseil-général*, 37.

35. Susan A. Crane notes that this commitment to crafting new narratives out of the material remains of the past amounted to "a new kind of completeness" later in the nineteenth century. *Collecting and Historical Consciousness in Early Nineteenth-Century Germany* (Ithaca, NY: Cornell University Press, 2000), 41.

36. "Monuments des beaux-arts," *Journal des arts, des sciences, et de littérature* 204 (30 floréal, year X [20 May 1802]: 265–70.

37. Lenoir, "Rapport d'Alexandre Lenoir au Comité de l'instruction publique tendant à la création du Musée des Monuments français au Dépot des Petits-Augustins" (18 July 1795), in *Archives du Musée des monuments français,* vol. 1, 29.

38. Lenoir, "Observations sur l'organisation du Musée des Monuments Français au jardin de Monceau" (23 October 1800), in *Archives du Musée des monuments français,* vol. 1, 196.

39. Lenoir, *MMF,* 8 vols. (Paris: Guilleminet, 1800–1821). Additionally, Lenoir published twelve editions of his *Description historique et chronologique des monuments de sculpture réunis au Musée des monuments français* (Paris, 1794–1815).

40. Tony Bennet refers to the things that complement or elaborate on museum narratives (guidebooks, captions, etc.) as a part of their "cultural frame." *The Birth of the Museum: History, Theory, Politics* (1995; reprint, London: Routledge, 2013), 131.

41. Lenoir, *MMF,* vol. 1 (1800), 50–51.

42. "Extrait des registres des délibérations du Comité d'instruction publique de la Convention nationale," 29 vendemiaire, year IV [21 October 1795], in *Archives du Musée des monuments français,* vol. 1, 34.

43. AN F17* 24 4 no. 28, Alexandre Lenoir to the Minister of the Interior, 28 fructidor, year IV [14 September 1796]. Also AN F17* 24 10 no. 47, Eloi Johanneau [Alexandre Lenoir], *Coup d'oeuil sur l'état actuel et future du musée des monuments français consacré a l'histoire de l'art en France* (Paris, 1809). Lenoir had good reason to be impressed with his work, since the Museum of French Monuments was the first institution of its kind. Although scholars attribute the first historically oriented museum display to the Dusseldorf Gallery in 1775, they tend to agree that Lenoir was the first to depict a specifically *national* history. Nikolaus Pevsner, *A History of Building Types* (Princeton, NJ: Princeton University Press, 1976). Similarly, Stephen Bann refers to the overall chronological scheme as "without precedent," in *The Clothing of Clio,* 83; and Stanley Mellon refers to the museum as one of the first "genuinely historical museums in the world," in "Alexandre Lenoir," 76.

44. Mercier, "Sur le dépôt des Petits-Augustins," 329.

45. Lenoir, *MMF,* vol. 1 (1800), 50.

46. AN F13 1113, Letter from Alexandre Lenoir to Jean-Antoine Chaptal, 18 pluviôse, year X [7 February 1802].

47. AN F17* 24 3, Alexandre Lenoir, "Revue des principaux monuments des différents siècles réunis dans le Musée des monuments français. Considérés particulièrement sous le rapport de l'histoire et des progrès de l'art en France."

48. Auguste von Kotzebue, *Travels from Berlin to Paris in the Year 1804* (London: R. Phillips, 1804), 3, 9–10.

49. Lenoir, *MMF,* vol. 1 (1800), 181.

50. Lenoir, *MMF,* vol. 3 (1802), 87.

51. Eyre, *Observations Made at Paris during the Peace,* 188.

52. McClellan, *Inventing the Louvre,* 190. Haskell makes a similar observation in *History and Its Images,* 242. Lenoir himself states this in *MMF,* vol. 1 (1800). A review of this book published anonymously in the *Mercure de France* vol. 23 (1 prairial, year IX [21 May 1801]) takes issue with this narrative.

53. Lenoir, *MMF,* vol. 3 (1802), 29.

54. Lenoir, *MMF*, vol. 5 (1806), 14–16.

55. Lenoir, *MMF*, vol. 2 (1801), xcix–cxxiv.

56. Ibid., lxxvi, cxx.

57. Ibid., cviii.

58. Ibid., cxv.

59. Lenoir, *MMF*, vol. 9 (1810), i.

60. Mercier, "Sur le dépôt des Petits-Augustins," 326.

61. Williams, *Sketches of the State of Manners and Opinions in the French Republic*, 226, 231, 232.

62. Anne Plumptre, *A Narrative of Three Years' Residence in France, Principally in the Southern Departments, from the Year 1802–1805* (London: J. Mawman, 1810), 32.

63. Yorke, *Letters from France*, 116.

64. Jules Michelet, *Histoire de la Révolution française*, 2nd ed. (Paris: Librairie internationale, 1869), 297.

65. Plumptre, *A Narrative of Three Years' Residence in France*, 34.

66. James Forbes, *Letters from France, Written in the Years 1803 and 1804*, vol. 1 (London: J. White, 1806), 406–7.

67. Louis Courajod, ed., *Alexandre Lenoir, son journal et le Musée des monuments français*, vol. 1 (Paris: Honoré-Champion, 1878), 107.

68. BNF YA2–151–8, Alexandre Lenoir, "Ancien musée des monuments français, crée en 1789, détruit en 1816," in *Recueil factice de coupures de presse. Articles d'Alexandre Lenoir, tome I: Articles parus dans le Journal des Artistes*, 129.

69. Architectural historians in particular have discussed this shift in sensibilities about spaces for the dead. Two classic, but still very relevant examples are Richard Etlin, *The Architecture of Death: The Transformation of the Cemetery in Eighteenth-century Paris* (Cambridge, MA: MIT Press, 1987); and Blanche M. G. Linden, *Silent City on a Hill: Picturesque Landscapes of Memory and Boston's Mount Auburn Cemetery* (Cambridge, MA: University of Massachusetts Press, 2007 [1989]).

70. Pierre Dolivier, *Essai sur les funérailles* (Versailles, year IX [1800–1801]), 59.

71. Martin Calder, "Promenade in Ermenonville," in *Experiencing the Garden in the Eighteenth Century*, ed. Martin Calder (Bern: Peter Lang, 2006), 109–44; Clarke, *Commemorating the Dead in Revolutionary France*, 13–22.

72. AN F17* 24 11, Letter from Alexandre Lenoir to the Minister of the Interior (Jean-Pierre Bachasson), 22 August 1813.

73. AN F17*24 3 no 147, Letter from citoyen Lesieur to citoyen Lenoir, 14 pluviôse, year IV [3 February 1796]. For more about the fate of Descartes's remains throughout history, see Russell Shorto, *Descartes's Bones: A Skeletal History of the Conflict between Faith and Reason* (New York: Doubleday, 2008).

74. Lenoir, *MMF*, vol. 5 (1806), 195, 200–202.

75. Lenoir was so concerned about accuracy that he had a mask of Héloïse's face made out of the remaining pieces of her skull, so that the figure laying on her tomb would most closely resemble her.

76. Lenoir, *MMF*, vol. 1 (1800), 224.

77. AN F17*24 6 no. 41, Letter from Alexandre Lenoir to the Minister of the Interior (Lucien Bonaparte), 24 pluviôse, year VIII [13 February 1800].

78. Charles Pye, *Rambles Abroad, or, Observations on the Continent, Made during the Summers of the Years 1816, 1817, 1818, in Excursions through Part of the North of France, the Low Countries, along the Rhine and the Prussian Frontier* (London: J. Carpenter & Son, 1823), 258.

79. Lenoir, *MMF,* vol. 1 (1801), 230–38.

80. AN F21 568, Letter from Alexandre Lenoir to the Minister of the Interior (Lucien Bonaparte), 24 pluviôse, year VIII [13 February 1800].

81. Lenoir, *MMF,* vol. 1 (1800), 219.

82. The quote that Lenoir indicates was inscribed on the inside of Coligny's mausoleum wrote that while Coligny's head was brought to his Medici opponents, his body was left for scavenging "ravenous birds." Lenoir, *MMF,* vol. 6 (1811), 292.

83. Ibid., 291.

84. Lenoir, *MMF,* vol. 4 (1805), 26–27.

85. Lenoir, *MMF,* vol. 1 (1800), 223–24.

86. Yorke, *Letters from France,* 129.

87. AN F17*24 12, Alexandre Lenoir, "Notice historique sur les sépultures d'Héloïse et d'Abélard" (1815).

88. AN F17*24 5 no. 24, Letter from Alexandre Lenoir to the Minister of the Interior (Nicolas-Louis François de Neufchâteau), 2 germinal, year VII [22 March 1799].

89. F17* 25 5 no. 32, Alexandre Lenoir's procès verbal, 15 floréal, year VIII [5 May 1800].

90. Ibid.

91. Lenoir, *MMF,* vol. 5 (1806), 201.

92. Lenoir, *MMF,* vol. 9 (1810), 277–84.

93. The two most notable examples of this trend are Marisa Linton, *Choosing Terror: Virtue, Friendship, and Authenticity in the French Revolution* (Oxford: Oxford University Press, 2015); and Sarah Horowitz, *Friendship and Politics in Post-Revolutionary France* (University Park: Penn State University Press, 2014).

94. AN F17*24 6 no. 41, Letter from Alexandre Lenoir to the Minister of the Interior (Lucien Bonaparte), 24 pluviôse, year VIII [13 February 1800].

95. Lenoir, *MMF,* vol. 5 (1806), 200.

96. Louis Courajod, ed., *Alexandre Lenoir, son journal et le Musée des monuments fran-çais,* vol. 2 (Paris: Honoré-Champion, 1878), 6.

97. AN F17* 24 8 no. 11, Letter from Bettencourt to Alexandre Lenoir, 22 ventôse, year VIII [25 February 1800].

98. AN F17*24 12 no. 35. In March 1816 the Prince de Condé reclaimed his ancestral property, including stained glass windows, busts, and mausoleums of Bourbon kings.

Conclusion: The Historian of the Dead

1. Jules Michelet, *Histoire de la Révolution française,* vol. 7 (Paris: Chamerot, 1853), 420.

2. Jules Michelet, *Histoire du XIXe siècle,* vol. 1 (Paris: Lévy, 1876), 129.

3. Jules Michelet, *Journal,* ed. Paul Viallaneix, vol. 1 (Paris: Gallimard, 1959), 116. Translation from *Mother Death: The Journal of Jules Michelet, 1815–1850,* trans. and ed. Edward K. Kaplan (Amherst: University of Massachusetts Press, 1984), 53–55.

4. Jules Michelet, *Mon journal, 1820–1823* (Paris: Flammarion, 1888), 172.

5. Michelet refers to bringing his manuscripts to Poinsot's gravesite on March 27, 1821. *Mon journal,* 181. This was the first, but not the last time that he brought work to the cemetery. See also ibid., 231, 238.

6. Ibid., 217, and *Journal,* vol. 1, 120, 220, 327.

7. Michelet, *Journal,* vol. 1, 328.

8. The first instance of this occurred on June 24, 1821, when he watered the flowers that were "dying of thirst" on some strangers' graves. Michelet, *Mon journal,* 217.

9. Ibid., 99.

10. Michelet, *Journal,* vol. 1, 120.

11. Ibid.

12. Ibid., 116. Several years later, in April 1842, Michelet similarly referred to Père Lachaise Cemetery as "the entire nineteenth century, accumulated in one place." Ibid., 395.

13. The first of Michelet's many volumes on his nation's history, *History of France*, vol. 1 (up to 1270) appeared in December 1833. He completed the last of his books about French history, vol. 3 of *History of the Nineteenth Century* in January 1874. He died less than a month later, on February 9.

14. Hédia Balafrej, "Alfred Dumesnil: Le jeune hôte de la rue des postes," *Dialogues autour de Vascoeuil: Dumesnil et Michelet*, ed. Paul Viallaneix and Simone Bernard Griffiths (Paris: Librairie Nizet, 1995), 35.

15. Jules Michelet, *Histoire de la Révolution française*, vol. 6 (Paris: Chamerot, 1853), 218.

16. Michelet quoted in Dominique Poulot, "Les musées d'histoire et la conscience nationale," *Archives et nations dans l'Europe du XIXe siècle*, ed. Bruno Delmas and Christine Nougaret (Paris: École des chartes, 2004), 198.

17. Jules Michelet, *Histoire de France*, new ed., vol. 3 (Paris: A. Le Vasseur, 1876), 232–33.

18. A good example of a postmodern scholar attempting to make sense of Michelet's relationship to this is Caroline Steedman, "Something She Called a Fever: Michelet, Derrida, and Dust," *American Historical Review* 106, no. 4 (October 2001): 1159–80.

19. Jules Michelet, *Histoire du XIXe siècle*, vol. 2 (Paris: Lévy, 1880), iv; Jules Michelet, "Préface de 1869," *Histoire de France*, new ed., vol. 1 (Paris: A. Le Vasseur, 1876), iii. For more on Michelet's approach to history, see chapters 1 and 3 in Roland Barthes, *Michelet*, trans. Richard Howard (New York: Hill & Wang, 1987), 17–25, 55–79.

20. The most obvious example of this is, of course, Michelet's *Le Peuple* (Paris: Hachette, 1846).

21. François Furet, *Interpreting the French Revolution*, trans. Elborg Forster (Cambridge: Cambridge University Press, 1981), 16.

BIBLIOGRAPHY

Archival Sources

Archives de l'Institut de France [AIF]

1H5, 1H6, 1H7

Archives Nationales de France [AN]

F1cl I87
F8 92
F13 203, F13 330, F13 524, F13 742, F13 908, F13 1113
F14 2728
F17 1280a
F17* 24, F17* 25
F19 4379

Archives de Paris [AP]

VD4 10

Bibliothèque Historique de la Ville de Paris [BHVP]

MSS 11

Bibliothèque Nationale de France [BNF]

Collection Joly de Fleury, 1209
Estampes et Photographes, YA2-151-8

Newspapers

Gazette nationale, ou le Moniteur universel
Journal de la montagne
Journal de Paris
Journal des débats et des décrets
Mercure de France
Les Révolutions de Paris
Revue de Paris

Published Primary Sources

Anon. "Monuments des beaux-arts." *Journal des arts, des sciences, et de la littérature* 204 (30 Floréal, year X [20 May 1802]): 265–270.

Anon. *Memorandums of a Residence in France, in the Winter of 1815–1816, Including Remarks on French Manners and Society, with a Description of the Catacombs, and Notices of Some Other Objects of Curiosity and Works of Art, not Hitherto Described.* London: Longman, Hurst, Rees, Orme, and Brown, 1816.

Anon. "Thury on the Catacombs of Paris." *British Review, and London Critical Journal* 7, no. 13 (1816): 125–145.

Anon. *Recherches statistiques sur la ville de Paris et le département de la Seine. Recueil de tableaux.* Paris: Imprimerie royale, 1826.

Anon. "Album." *Revue des deux mondes, journal des voyages, des sciences, de l'administration, des moeurs, etc . . . chez les différents peuples du globe, par une société de savants* 2, no. 2 (1830): 417–426.

Arnaud, C.-P. *Recueil de tombeaux des quatre cimetières de Paris, avec leurs épitaphes et leurs inscriptions.* 2 vols. Paris: Arnaud, Mathiot, Carillan-Goeury, Delaunay, 1817–1825.

Avril, Jean-Baptiste. *Rapport de l'administration des travaux publics, sur les cimetières, lu au conseil-général par le citoyen Avril.* Paris, 1794.

Barrère, Bertrand. *Rapport fait au nom du comité du salut public, le premier août 1793, l'an II de la République Française.* Paris: Imprimerie nationale, 1793.

Batissier, L. *Histoire de Paris et de ses monuments, nouvelle édition refondue et complété jusqu'à nos jours.* Paris: Furne, 1846.

Bayard, H. "Mémoire sur la police des cimetières." *Annales d'hygiène publique et de médecine légale* 17 (1837): 196–309.

Berthet, Elie. *Les Catacombes de Paris*. Paris, 1854.

Bonnaffé, Edmond. "Les Restes d'un grand homme." *Gazette des beaux-arts* 27 (April 1883): 324–326.

Brogniart, Alexandre-Théodore. *Plans du palais de la Bourse de Paris, et du cimetière Mont-Louis en six planches*. Paris: Crapelet, 1814.

Cadet de Vaux, Antoine-Alexis. "Mémoire historique et physique sur le cimetière des Innocents." *Journal de Physique* 22 (June 1783): 409–417.

Caillot, Antoine. *Voyage religieux et sentimentale aux quatre cimetières de Paris*. Paris, 1809.

Caillot, Antoine. *Mémoire pour servir à l'histoire des moeurs et usages des Français, depuis les plus hautes conditions jusqu'aux classes inférieures de la société, pendant le règne de Louis XVI, sous le Directoire exécutive, sous Napoléon Bonaparte, et jusqu'à nos jours*. 2 vols. Paris: Dauvin, 1827.

Cambry, Jacques. *Rapport sur les sépultures: Présenté à l'administration centrale du département de la Seine*. Paris, year VII (1799–1800).

du Camp, Maxime. *Paris, ses organes, ses fonctions, et sa vie dans la seconde moitié du XIXe siècle*. 6 vols. Paris: Hachette, 1875.

de Chateaubriand, René. *The Genius of Christianity*. Translated by Charles White. Baltimore: John Murphy, 1856.

de Chateaubriand, René. *Mémoires d'outre-tombe*. 6 vols. Paris: Dufour, Mulat, et Boulanger, 1860.

Coindre, Jean-Jacques. *Mémoire sur la translation des cimetières hors de la ville de Lyon*. Lyon, 1789.

Collection des lois, senatus-consultes, décrets impériaux et avis du conseil d'état relatifs aux cultes; publiés depuis le Concordat jusqu'au 1er janvier 1813 inclusivement. Paris: Rivals, 1813.

[Colnet du Ravel, Charles Joseph]. *L'Hermite du faubourg Saint-Germain, ou observations sur les moeurs et les usages français au commencement du XIXe siècle*. Paris: Pillet aîné, 1825.

Coupé, Jean-Marie. *Des sépultures en politique et en morale*. Paris: Imprimerie nationale, 1796.

Coupé, Jean-Marie. *De la moralité des sépultures et de leur police*. Paris: C. Vollant, 1800.

Courajod, Louis, ed. *Alexandre Lenoir, son journal et le Musée des monuments français*. 3 vols. Paris: Honoré-Champion, 1878–1887.

Daubermesnil, François-Antoine. *Corps législatif. Conseil des cinq-cents. Rapport sur les inhumations. Séance du 21 Brumaire an V*. Paris: Imprimerie nationale, year V (1796–1797).

Delamalle, Gaspard-Gilbert. *Réflexions sur l'enterrement de ma mère: Ou, sur les cérémonies et la moralité des institutions civiles en générale*. 2nd ed. Paris: Librairie Chrétienne, year IV (1795–1796).

Détruisard, Thomas. *Essai sur les Catacombes de Paris*. Paris, 1812.

Doderet, Thomas. *Catéchisme de toutes les religions en abrégé, dédié au Cercle constitutionnel de la commune de Langres*. Chaumont: Imprimerie de Cousot, year VI (1797–1798).

Dolivier, Pierre. *Essai sur les funérailles.* Versailles: Jacob, year X (1800–1801).

Dulaure, Jacques-Antoine. *Histoire physique, civile, et morale de Paris: depuis les premiers temps historiques jusqu'à nos jours* [. . .] *ornée de gravures représentant divers plan de Paris, ses monuments et édifices principaux.* 2nd ed. 10 vols. Paris: Guillaume, 1823–1824.

Dulaure, Jacques-Antoine. *Panorama de la ville de Paris et guide de l'étranger à Paris.* Paris: P.-Corneille, 1824.

Dumas, Alexandre. *Les Mohicans de Paris.* 4 vols. Paris: Michel Lévy frères, 1871–1872.

Eyre, Edmund John. *Observations Made at Paris during the Peace.* London: W. Meyler, 1803.

de Feller, F-X., Charles Weiss, and l'abbé Busson. *Biographie universelle, ou, dictionnaire historique des hommes qui se sont fait un nom par leur génie, leurs talents, leurs vertus, leurs erreurs ou leurs crimes.* 10 vols. Paris: Gaume Frères, 1848.

Frochot, Nicolas. *Arrêté du préfet du département de la Seine concernant les inhumations.* Paris, 1801.

Géraud, Edmond. *Journal d'un étudiant pendant la Révolution, 1789–1795.* Edited by Gaston Maugras. Paris: Calmann Lévy, 1890.

G.G. *Promenade sérieuse au cimetière du Père La Chaise, ou de Mont-Louis, près de Paris.* Paris: Imprimerie de Lachevardière fils, 1826.

de Girard, Joseph. *Des Tombeaux: Ou, de l'influence des institutions funèbres sur les moeurs.* Paris: F. Buisson, 1801.

Giraud, Pierre. *Pétition du citoyen Giraud, ci-devant Architecte du département de Paris, à la convention nationale.* Paris: Veuve Hérissant, 1794.

Giraud, Pierre. *Essai sur les sépultures: Composé en l'an 4, et déposé au département de la Seine, le 11 nivôse, an 7, avec les plans, coupes, et élévations du monument projeté.* Paris: R. Jacquin, 1799.

Giraud, Pierre. *Les Tombeaux, ou essai sur les sépultures. Ouvrage dans lequel l'auteur rappelle les coutumes des anciens peuples; cite sommairement celles observées par les modernes; donne les procédés pour dissoudre les chairs, calciner les ossements humains, les convertir en une substance indestructible, et en composer le médaillon de chaque individu.* 2nd ed. Paris: Desenne, 1801.

Grégoire, Henri. *Rapport sur les destructions opérées par le vandalisme, et sur les moyens de le réprimer . . . Suivi du décret de la Convention nationale.* Paris: Imprimerie nationale, 1794.

Griscom, John. *A Year in Europe: Comparing a Journal of Observations in England, Scotland, Ireland, France, Switzerland, and the North of Italy, and Holland. In 1818 and 1819.* 2 vols. New York: Collins & Co., 1824.

de Guilhermy, Le Bon. *Monographie de l'Église royale de Saint-Denis: tombeaux et figures historiques.* Paris: V. Didron, 1848.

Guillon, Aimé. *Les Martyrs de la foi pendant la Révolution française, ou, Martyrologie des pontifs, prêtres, religieux, religieuses, laïcs de l'un et l'autre sexe, qui périrent alors pour la foi.* Paris: G. Mathiot, 1821.

Guillon, Marie-Nicolas-Silvestre [Le C . . .]. *Sur le respect dû aux tombeaux; et l'indécence des inhumations actuelles. Nouvelle édition, augmentée de la sépulture et de la mélancolie, poèmes de Legouvé.* Paris, year VIII (1799–1800).

H., T. "Fragments Illustrative of Paris, in 1814: The Catacombs." *New Monthly Magazine and Universal Register* 22 (November 1, 1815): 308–312.

Hallé, Desessartz, Toulogeon, Reviellère-Lepaux, Leblond, and Camus. *Rapport fait par les citoyens Hallé, Desessartz, Toulogeon, Reviellère-Lepaux, Leblond et Camus, commissaires chargés par l'Institut nationale des Sciences et Arts, de l'examen des mémoires envoyés au concours proposé par le gouvernement, sur les questions relatives aux cérémonies funéraires et aux lieux des sépultures. Jugement porté par l'Institut et proclamation du prix.* Paris: Bailleul, 1800.

d'Heilly, Georges. *Extraction des cercueils royaux à Saint-Denis en 1793.* Paris: Hachette, 1868.

Héricart de Thury, Louis-Etienne. *Description des Catacombes de Paris précédée d'un précis historique sur les catacombes de tous les peuples de l'ancien et du nouveau continent.* Paris, 1815. Reprinted with preface by Marc Viré. Paris: CTHS, 2005.

de Jolimont, F.-G.-T. *Les Mausolées français: recueil des tombeaux les plus remarquables par leur structure, leurs épitaphes ou les cendres qu'ils contiennent, érigés dans les nouveaux cimetières de Paris.* Paris: Firmin-Didot, 1821.

[de Jouy, Etienne]. *L'Hermite de la Chaussée-d'Antin, ou, observations sur les moeurs et les usages parisiennes au commencement du XIXe siècle.* Vol. 2. Paris: Pilet, 1812–1814.

von Kotzebue, Auguste. *Travels from Berlin to Paris in the Year 1804.* London: R. Phillips, 1804.

LaFargue, Jean-Baptiste. *Motion d'ordre sur la police des cimetières et des inhumations.* Paris: Imprimerie nationale, year VII (1798–1799).

de Lamarque, Nestor. *Trois élégies.* Paris: Les Librairies du Palais-royal, 1824.

de Lamarque, Nestor. "Les Catacombes de Paris." In *Paris, ou le livre des cent et un.* Vol. 6. 19–34. Paris: Ladvocat, 1832.

Legouvé, Gabriel-Marie. *Les Souvenirs, la Sépulture et la Mélancolie.* Paris: Lemierre, year VI (1797–1798).

Lenoir, Alexandre. *Notice succincte des objets de sculpture et architecture réunis au dépôt provisoire national, rue des Petits-Augustins.* Paris: Desenne, 1793.

Lenoir, Alexandre. *Notice historique des monuments des arts réunis au dépot national; rue des Petits Augustins au ci-devant couvent de la reine Marguerite.* Paris: Desenne, 1795.

Lenoir, Alexandre. *Description historique et chronologique des monuments de sculpture réunis au Musée des monuments français [. . .].* 10 vols. Paris, 1797–1816.

Lenoir, Alexandre. *Musée des monuments français, ou Description historique et chronologique des statues en marbre et en bronze, bas-reliefs, et tombeaux des hommes et femmes célèbres, pour servir à l'histoire de France et à celle de l'art, ornée de gravures et augmentée d'une dissertation sur le costume de chaque siècle.* 8 vols. Paris: Guilleminet, 1800–1821.

[Lenoir, Alexandre] Johanneau, Eloi (pseud.). *Coup d'oeuil sur l'état actuel et future du Musée des monuments français consacré à l'histoire de l'art en France.* Paris, 1809.

M**** [pseud.]. *Le Cimetière de la Madeleine.* Paris, 1800.

Marchant de Beaumont, François-Marie. *Le Conducteur de l'étranger à Paris.* Paris, 1815.

Marchant de Beaumont, François-Marie. *Le Conducteur au cimetière de l'est, ou du Père La Chaise; contenant l'esquisse descriptive et topographique de ce lieu funèbre, et le tableau des scènes de moeurs dont il est le témoin.* Paris: Plassan, 1820.

Marchant de Beaumont, François-Marie. *Vues pittoresques, historiques, et morales du cimetière du P. La Chaise. Dessinée par MM. Vigneront et Duplat, et gravées à l'aqua-tinta par M. Jazet et les meilleurs artistes.* Paris, 1821.

Mercier, Louis-Sébastien. *Tableau de Paris.* 8 vols. Amsterdam, 1783–1789.

Mercier, Louis-Sébastien. "Sur le dépôt des Petits-Augustins, dit: le Musée des monuments français." *Journal d'économie publique, de morale, et de politique* 5 (1797): 325–329.

Méry, Joseph. *Salons et souterrains de Paris.* Paris: Schiller, 1851.

Michelet, Jules. *Le Peuple.* Paris: Hachette, 1846.

Michelet, Jules. *Histoire de la Révolution française.* 7 vols. Paris: Chamerot, 1847–1853.

Michelet, Jules. *Histoire du XIXe siècle.* 3 vols. Paris: Lévy, 1875–1876.

Michelet, Jules. *Histoire de France.* New ed. 19 vols. Paris: A. Le Vasseur, 1876–1878.

Michelet, Jules. *Mon journal, 1820–1823.* Paris: Flammarion, 1888.

Michelet, Jules. *Journal; texte intégral, établi sur les manuscrits autographes et publié pour la première fois, avec une introduction, des notes et de nombreux documents inédits.* Edited by Paul Viallaneix. 2 vols. Paris: Gallimard, 1959–1962.

Ministère de l'instruction publique et des beaux-arts. *Inventaire général des richesses d'art de la France. Archives du musée des monuments français.* 3 vols. Paris: E. Plon, 1883–1897. Facsimile of the original. Elibron Classics, 2005.

de Moy, Charles-Alexandre. *Accord de la religion et des cultes chez une nation libre.* Paris: J.-B. Garnéry, 1792.

Mulot, François-Valentin. *Vues d'un citoyen, ancien député de Paris à l'Assemblée législative, sur les sépultures.* Paris: Imprimerie de la rue des Droits de l'homme, 1797.

Nadar, Félix. "Le Dessus et le dessous de Paris." In *Paris guide, par les principaux écrivains et artistes de la France.* Vol. 2. *La vie.* 1569–1591. Paris: A. Lacroix, 1867.

Pastoret, Emmanuel. *Rapport sur la violation des sépultures et des tombeaux, fait aux nom de la commission de la classification et de la révision des lois.* Paris: Imprimerie nationale, year IV (1795–1796).

[Piétresson de Saint-Aubin, Pierre] M. P. St.-A. *Promenade aux cimetières de Paris, aux sépultures royales de Saint-Denis, et aux Catacombes [. . .].* Paris: Panckoucke, 1816.

Pillet, Fabien. "Vers faits dans les Catacombes de Paris." *Almanach des muses* 55 (1819): 208.

Plumptre, Anne. *A Narrative of Three Years' Residence in France, Principally in the Southern Departments, from the Year 1802–1805: Including Some Authentic Particulars Respecting the Early Life of the French Emperor, and a General Inquiry into his Character.* London: J. Mawman, 1810.

Pommereul, [François-René-Jean] Général. *Mémoire sur les funérailles. Question proposée par le Ministère, et jugée par l'Institut, le 15 vendémiaire, an IX.* Tours: Billault jeune, year IX (1800–1801).

Pye, Charles. *Rambles Abroad, or, Observations on the Continent, Made during the Summers of the Years 1816, 1817, 1818, in Excursions through Part of the North of France, the Low Countries, along the Rhine and the Prussian Frontier.* London: J. Carpenter & Son, 1823.

Quatremère de Quincy, Antoine. *Rapport fait au Conseil-Général; le 15 thermidor, an VIII, sur l'Instruction publique, le rétablissement des bourses, le scandale des inhumations actuelles, l'érection de cimetières, la restitution des tombeaux, mausolées, etc.* Paris: R. Jacquin, year 8 (1799–1800).

Quatremère de Quincy, Antoine. *Considérations morales sur la destination des ouvrages de l'art.* Paris: Crapelet, 1815.

Raunier, Emile, ed. *Épitaphier du vieux Paris: Recueil général des inscriptions funéraires des églises, couvents, collèges, hospices, cimetières et charniers, depuis le moyen âge jusqu'à la fin du XVIIIe siècle.* 3 vols. Paris, 1890–1901.

Roederer, Pierre-Louis. *Des institutions funéraires convenables a une république qui permet tous les cultes, et n'adopte aucun: mémoire lu par Roederer, dans la séance publique de l'Institut national des Sciences et des Arts, le 25 Messidor, l'an IV.* Paris: B. Mathey, 1796.

Roger, M. M. [father and son]. *Le Champ du repos, ou le cimetière Mont-Louis dit du Père Lachaise, ouvrage orné avec de planches, représentant plus de 2000 mausolées érigés dans ce cimetière, depuis sa création jusqu'au 1er janvier, 1816, avec leurs épitaphes; son plan topographique, te qu'il existait du temps du père delachaise, et tel qu'il existe aujourd'hui; précédé du portrait de ce jésuite, d'un abrégé de sa vie; et suivi de quelques remarques sur la manière dont différens peuples honorent les défunts.* 2 vols. Paris: Pillet, 1816.

Ronesse, A.-J. *Projet pour les sépultures.* Paris: Debray, year IX (1800–1801).

Sade, D. A. F. *Idées sur les romans.* Edited by Octave Uzanne. Paris: Edouard Rouveyre, 1878.

Scott, John. *A Visit to Paris in 1814: Being a Review of the Moral, Political, Intellectual, and Social Condition of the French Capital.* Philadelphia: Edward Parker, 1815.

Stevenson, Seth Williams. *Journal of a Tour through Part of France, Flanders, and Holland, including a Visit to Paris, and a Walk over the Field of Waterloo: Made in the Summer of 1816.* Norwich: Norfolk Chronicle Press, 1817.

Thiébaut, Arsenne. *Réflexions sur les pompes funèbres.* Paris: Galetti, year IV (1797–1798).

Thiessé, Léon. *Les Catacombes de Paris, poème en un chant.* Paris: Hocquet, 1815.

Thouret, Michel-Augustin. *Rapport sur les exhumations du cimetière et de l'église des SS Innocens: Lu dans la séance royale de médecine, tenue au Louvre, le 3 mars 1789.* Paris: P.-D. Pierres, 1789.

Vaudoyer, Jean-Louis. *Idées d'un citoyen sur le lieu destiné à la sépulture des hommes illustres de France.* Paris, 1791.

Villedieu. *Projet de catacombes pour la ville de Paris en adaptant à cet usage les carrières qui se trouvent tant dans son enceinte que dans ses environs.* Paris, 1782.

Warin, J. G. *Le Cimetière de la Madeleine.* Paris: Le Petit Jeune, 1800.

Willermoz, Dutreih, Roux, and Carret. *Les Commissaires aux inhumations, aux citoyens maire et officiers municipaux de Commune-Affranchie.* Lyon: Imprimerie républicaine, 1794.

Williams, Helena Maria. *Sketches of the State of Manners and Opinions in the French Republic, towards the Close of the Eighteenth Century.* London: G. G. and J. Robinson, 1801.

Yorke, Henry Redhead. *Letters from France, in 1802.* London: H. D. Symonds, 1804.

Zaccone, Pierre. *Les Drames des catacombes.* Paris: Ballay aîné, 1863.

Secondary Sources

Alexander, Robert. *Re-writing the French Revolution Tradition: Liberal Opposition and the Fall of the Bourbon Monarchy.* Cambridge: Cambridge University Press, 2004.

Alpaugh, Micah. *Non-violence and the French Revolution: Political Demonstrations in Paris, 1787–1795.* Cambridge: Cambridge University Press, 2015.

Andress, David. *The Terror: The Merciless War for Freedom in Revolutionary France.* New York: Farrar, Straus & Giroux, 2005.

Arasse, Daniel. *The Guillotine and the Terror.* Translated by Christopher Miller. London: Allen Lane, 1989.

Ariès, Philippe. *The Hour of Our Death.* Translated by Helen Weaver. New York: Knopf, 1981.

Armenteros, Carolina. *The French Idea of History: Joseph de Maistre and His Heirs, 1794–1854.* Ithaca, NY: Cornell University Press, 2011.

Aston, Nigel. *Religion and Revolution in France 1780–1804.* Washington, D.C.: Catholic University Press, 2000.

Aulard, François Alphonse. *Le culte de la raison et le culte de l'être suprême, 1793–1794: Essai historique.* Paris: F. Alcan, 1892.

Baczko, Bronislaw. *Ending the Terror: The French Revolution after Robespierre.* Translated by Michel Petheram. Cambridge: Cambridge University Press, 1994.

de Baecque, Antoine. *Glory and Terror: Seven Deaths under the French Revolution.* Translated by Charlotte Mandell. New York: Routledge, 2001.

Balafrej, Hédia. "Alfred Dumesnil: Le jeune hôte de la rue des postes." In *Dialogues autour de Vascoeuil: Dumesnil et Michelet,* edited by Paul Viallaneix and Simone Bernard Griffiths, 27–43. Paris: Librairie Nizet, 1995.

Bann, Stephen. *The Clothing of Clio: A Study of the Representation of History in Nineteenth-Century Britain and France.* Cambridge: Cambridge University Press, 1984.

Bann, Stephen. *Romanticism and the Rise of History.* New York: Twayne, 1995.

Barnes, David S. *The Great Stink of Paris and the Nineteenth-Century Struggle against Filth and Germs.* Baltimore: Johns Hopkins University Press, 2006.

Barthes, Roland. *Michelet.* Translated by Richard Howard. New York: Hill & Wang, 1987.

Bauchal, Charles. *Nouveau dictionnaire biographique et critique des architectes français.* Paris: Librairie générale de l'architecture, 1887.

Bell, David A. *The Cult of the Nation in France: Inventing Nationalism, 1680–1800.* Cambridge, MA: Harvard University Press, 2003.

Ben-Amos, Avner. *Funerals, Politics, and Memory in Modern France, 1789–1996.* Oxford: Oxford University Press, 2000.

Bennet, Tony. *The Birth of the Museum: History, Theory, Politics.* London: Routledge, 1995.

Bergdoll, Barry, ed. *Le Panthéon: Symbole des revolutions.* Paris: Picard, 1989.

Bertrand, Régis. "L'invention du cimetière français contemporain au Père-Lachaise au début du XIXe siècle." *Annales de l'Est* 2 (2012): 185–203.

Bonnet, Jean-Claude. *Naissance du Panthéon: Essai sur le culte des grands hommes.* Paris: Fayard, 1998.

Bossut, Nicole. "Aux origines de la déchristianisation dans le Nièvre: Fouché, Chaumette, ou les jacobins nivernais?" *Annales historiques de la Révolution française* 264 (1986): 181–202. https://doi.org/10.3406/ahrf.1986.1167.

Boudon, Jacques-Olivier. *Napoléon et les cultes: Les religions en Europe à l'aube du XIXe siècle (1800–1815).* Paris: Fayard, 2002.

Bouwers, Eveline. *Public Pantheons in Revolutionary Europe: Comparing Cultures, c. 1790–1840.* New York: Palgrave, 2012.

Brooks, Peter. *The Melodramatic Imagination: Balzac, Henry James, Melodrama, and the Mode of Excess.* New Haven, CT: Yale University Press, 1995.

Brown, Howard. *Ending the Revolution: Violence, Justice, and Repression from the Terror to Napoleon.* Charlottesville: University of Virginia Press, 2006.

Brown, Howard G., and Judith A. Miller, eds. *Taking Liberties: Problems of a New Order from the French Revolution to Napoleon.* Manchester: Manchester University Press, 2002.

Burton, June K. *Napoleon and the Woman Question: Discourses of the Other Sex in French Education, Medicine, and Medical Law, 1799–1815.* Lubbock: Texas Tech University Press, 2007.

Calder, Martin, ed. *Experiencing the Garden in the Eighteenth Century.* Bern: Peter Lang, 2006.

Chaunu, Pierre. *La Mort à Paris 16e, 17e, 18e siècles.* Paris: Fayard, 1978.

Clarke, Joseph. *Commemorating the Dead in Revolutionary France: Revolution and Remembrance, 1789–1799.* Cambridge: Cambridge University Press, 2007.

Cohen, William A., and Ryan Johnson, eds. *Filth: Dirt, Disgust, and Modern Life.* Minneapolis: University of Minnesota Press, 2005.

Corbin, Alain. *The Foul and the Fragrant: Odor and the French Social Imagination.* Cambridge, MA: Harvard University Press, 1988.

Crane, Susan A. *Collecting and Historical Consciousness in Early Nineteenth-Century Germany.* Ithaca, NY: Cornell University Press, 2000.

Davidson, Denise Z. *France after Revolution: Urban Life, Gender, and the New Social Order.* Cambridge, MA: Harvard University Press, 2007.

Denby, David. *Sentimental Narrative and the Social Order in France, 1760–1820.* Cambridge: Cambridge University Press, 1994.

Dommanget, Maurice, and Michel Vovelle, *Enragés et curés rouges en 1793: Jacques Roux, Pierre Dolivier.* Paris: Spartacus, 1993.

Etlin, Richard. "The Cemetery and the City: Paris, 1744–1804." Ph.D. diss, Princeton University, 1978. ProQuest (7818328).

Etlin, Richard. *The Architecture of Death: The Transformation of the Cemetery in Eighteenth-Century Paris.* Cambridge, MA: MIT Press, 1984.

Etlin, Richard. *Symbolic Space: French Enlightenment Architecture and Its Legacy.* Chicago: University of Chicago Press, 1994.

Ferguson, Priscilla. *Paris as Revolution: Writing the Nineteenth-Century City.* Berkeley: University of California Press, 1994.

Foisil, Madeleine. "Les attitudes devant la mort aux XVIIIe siècle: sépultures et suppressions de sépultures dans le cimetière parisien des Saints-Innocents." *Revue Historique* 251 (April–June 1974): 303–330. http://www.jstor.org/stable/40953030.

Forbes, James. *Letters from France, Written in the Years 1803 and 1804. Including a Particular Account of Verdun, and the Situation of the Captives in That City.* 2 vols. London: J. White, 1806.

Foucault, Michel. *The Order of Things: An Archaeology of the Human Sciences.* New York: Vintage, 1970.

Foucault, Michel. "Of Other Spaces." Translated by Jay Miskowiec. *Diacritics: A Review of Contemporary Criticism* 16, no. 1 (spring 1986): 22–27. http://www.jstor.org/stable/464648.

Fritzsche, Peter. *Stranded in the Present: Modern Time and the Melancholy of History.* Cambridge, MA: Harvard University Press, 2004.

Fureix, Emmanuel. *La France des larmes: deuils politiques à l'âge romantique, 1814–1840.* Seyssel: Champ Vallon, 2009.

Furet, François. *Interpreting the French Revolution.* Translated by Elborg Forster. Cambridge: Cambridge University Press, 1981.

Garrioch, David. *The Making of Revolutionary Paris.* Berkeley: University of California Press, 2004.

Gérards, Émile. *Les Catacombes de Paris.* Paris: Chamuel, 1892.

Greene, Christopher. "Alexandre Lenoir and the Musée des monuments français during the French Revolution." *French Historical Studies* 12, no. 2 (autumn 1981): 200–222. http://www.jstor.org/stable/286477.

Greybill, Lela. *The Visual Culture of Violence after the French Revolution.* New York: Routledge, 2016.

Goldhammer, Jesse. *The Headless Republic.* Ithaca, NY: Cornell University Press, 2005.

Goldstein, Jan. *The Post-Revolutionary Self: Politics and Psyche in France, 1750–1850.* Cambridge, MA: Harvard University Press, 2005.

Hannaway, Owen and Caroline. "Le fermeture du cimetière des Innocents." *Dix-huitième siècle* 9 (1977): 181–191. https://doi.org/10.3406/dhs.1977.1124.

Harding, Vanessa. *The Dead and the Living in Paris and London, 1500–1670.* Cambridge: Cambridge University Press, 2002.

Haskell, Francis. *History and Its Images: Art and the Interpretation of the Past.* New Haven, CT: Yale University Press, 1993.

Healey, Katherine, Karen Bowie, and Agnès Bos, eds. *Le Père Lachaise.* Paris: Action artistique de la ville de Paris, 1998.

Heuer, Jennifer. *The Family and the Nation: Gender and Citizenship in Revolutionary France.* Ithaca, NY: Cornell University Press, 2005.

Hintermeyer, Pascal. *Politiques de la mort: Tirées du concours de l'Institut, germinal an VIII–vendémiaire an IX.* Paris: Payot, 1981.

Horowitz, Sarah. *Friendship and Politics in Post-Revolutionary France.* University Park: Penn State University Press, 2013.

Hunt, David. "The People and Pierre Dolivier: Popular Uprisings in the Seine-et-Oise Department (1791–1792)." *French Historical Studies* 11, no. 2 (autumn 1979): 184–214. http://www.jstor.org/stable/i212705.

Hutton, Patrick H. *The Cult of the Revolutionary Tradition: The Blanquists in French Politics, 1864–1893.* Berkeley: University of California Press, 1981.

Hutton, Patrick H. *Philippe Ariès and the Politics of French Cultural History.* Amherst: University of Massachusetts Press, 2004.

Iverson, John. "Introduction to the Forum: Emulation in France, 1750–1800." *Eighteenth-Century Studies* 36, no. 2 (2003): 217–223. http://www.jstor.org/stable/30053361.

Jainchill, Andrew. *Reimagining Politics after the Terror: The Republican Origins of French Liberalism.* Ithaca, NY: Cornell University Press, 2008.

Jourdan, Annie. *Les Monuments de la Révolution, 1770–1804: Une histoire de representation.* Paris: Champion, 1997.

Kalifa, Dominique. "Crime Scenes: Criminal Topography and Social Imaginary in Nineteenth-Century Paris." Translated by Martine Andreoli. *French Historical Studies* 27, no. 1 (winter 2004): 175–194. https://doi.org/10.1215/00161071-27-1-175.

Kaplan, Edward K., ed. and trans. *Mother Death: The Journal of Jules Michelet, 1815–1850.* Amherst: University of Massachusetts Press, 1984.

Kaplan, Nira. "Virtuous Competition among Citizens: Emulation in Politics and Pedagogy during the French Revolution." *Eighteenth-Century Studies* 36, no. 2 (2003): 245–246. https://doi.org/10.1353/ecs.2003.0015.

Kingston, Ralph. *Bureaucrats and Bourgeois Society: Office Politics and Individual Credit in France, 1789–1848.* New York: Palgrave Macmillan, 2012.

Koselleck, Reinhart. *Future's Past: On the Semantics of Historical Time.* Translated by Keith Tribe. New York: Columbia University Press, 1985.

Koslofsky, Craig. *The Reformation of the Dead: Death and Ritual in Early Modern Germany, 1450–1700.* New York: St. Martin's Press, 2000.

Kroen, Sheryl. *Politics and Theatre: The Crisis of Legitimacy in Restoration France, 1815–1830.* Berkeley: University of California Press, 2000.

Kselman, Thomas. "The Dechristianization of Death in Modern France." In *The Decline of Christianity in Modern Europe*, edited by Hugh McLeod, 145–162. Cambridge: Cambridge University Press, 2004.

Laqueur, Thomas. "The Places of the Dead in Modernity." In *The Age of Cultural Revolutions in Britain and France, 1750–1820*, edited by Colin Jones and Dror Wahrman, 17–32. Berkeley: University of California Press, 2002.

Laqueur, Thomas. *The Work of the Dead: A Cultural History of Mortal Remains.* Princeton, NJ: Princeton University Press, 2015.

LaGlande, Vincent. *Histoire du Père Lachaise.* Paris: Vermet, 1988.

Lassère, Madeleine. *Villes et cimetières en France de l'Ancien Régime à nos jours.* Paris: Éditions l'Harmattan, 1997.

Lefebvre, Henri. *The Production of Space.* Translated by Donald Nicholson-Smith. Oxford: Wiley-Blackwell, 1992.

Linden, Blanche M. G. *Silent City on a Hill: Picturesque Landscapes of Memory and Boston's Mount Auburn Cemetery*. Rev. ed. Cambridge: University of Massachusetts Press, 2007.

Lindsay, Suzanne Glover. *Funerary Arts and Tomb Cult: Living with the Dead in France, 1750–1870*. Burlington, VT: Ashgate, 2012.

Lindsay, Suzanne Glover. "The Revolutionary Exhumations at St-Denis, 1793." *Conversations: An Online Journal of the Center for the Study of Material and Visual Cultures of Religion* (2014). doi:10.22332/con.ess.2015.2.

Linton, Marisa. *Choosing Terror: Virtue, Friendship, and Authenticity in the French Revolution*. Oxford: Oxford University Press, 2015.

Livesey, James. *Making Democracy in the French Revolution*. Cambridge, MA: Harvard University Press, 2012.

Lucas, Colin. "Revolutionary Violence." In *The French Revolution and the Creation of Modern Political Culture*, vol. 4, *The Terror*, edited by Keith Michael Baker, 57–79. Oxford: Pergamon Press, 1994.

Mah, Harold. *Enlightenment Phantasies: Cultural Identity in France and Germany, 1750–1914*. Ithaca, NY: Cornell University Press, 2003.

Maleuvre, Didier. *Museum Memories: History, Technology, Art*. Stanford, CA: Stanford University Press, 1999.

Martin, Jean-Clement. *Violence et Révolution: Essai sur la naissance d'un mythe national*. Paris: Éditions de Seuil, 2006.

Mason, Laura. "Never Was a Plot So Holy: Gracchus Babeuf and the End of the French Revolution." In *Conspiracy and the French Revolution*, edited by Thomas Kaiser, Marisa Linton, and Peter Campbell, 172–188. Manchester: Manchester University Press, 2007.

Mason, Laura. "The Culture of Reaction: Demobilizing the People after Thermidor." *French Historical Studies* 30, no. 3 (August 2016): 445–470. https://doi.org/10.1215/00161071-3500273.

Maza, Sarah. *The Myth of the French Bourgeoisie: An Essay on the Social Imaginary*. Cambridge, MA: Harvard University Press, 2003.

McClellan, Andrew. *Inventing the Louvre: Art, Politics, and the Origins of the Modern Museum in Eighteenth-Century Paris*. Cambridge: Cambridge University Press, 1994.

McManners, John. *The French Revolution and the Church*. New York: Harper & Row, 1970.

McManners, John. *Death and the Enlightenment: Changing Attitudes to Death among Christians and Unbelievers in Eighteenth-century France*. Oxford: Oxford University Press, 1981.

Mellon, Stanley. "Alexandre Lenoir: The Museum versus the Revolution." *Proceedings of the Consortium on Revolutionary Europe, 1750–1850* 9 (1979): 75–91.

Métayer, Christine. "Une espace de vie: les charniers du cimetière des SS. Innocents à Paris, sous l'Ancien Régime." *Journal of the Canadian Historical Association* 4, no. 1 (1993): 183–206. doi:10.7202/031062ar.

Naginski, Erika. *Sculpture and Enlightenment*. Los Angeles: The Getty Research Institute, 2009.

Ozouf, Mona. "Le Panthéon: L'école normale des morts." In *Les lieux de mémoire*, vol. 1, edited by Pierre Nora, 139–166. Paris: Gallimard, 1984.

Ozouf, Mona. *Festivals and the French Revolution*. Translated by Alan Sheridan. Cambridge, MA: Harvard University Press, 1988.

Perovic, Sanja. *The Calendar in Revolutionary France: Perceptions of Time in Literature, Culture, Politics*. Cambridge: Cambridge University Press, 2012.

Pevsner, Nikolaus. *A History of Building Types*. Princeton, NJ: Princeton University Press, 1976.

Pike, David Lawrence. "Paris Souterrain: Before and After the Revolution." *Dix-Neuf* 15, no. 2 (2011): 177–197. https://doi.org/10.1179/147873111X13113768737190.

Pilbeam, Pamela. *Madame Tussaud and the History of the Waxworks*. London: Hambledon & London, 2003.

Potofsky, Alan. *Constructing Paris in the Age of Revolution*. London: Palgrave Macmillan, 2009.

Poulot, Dominique. *Musée, nation, patrimoine (1789–1815)*. Paris: Gallimard, 1997.

Poulot, Dominique. "The Birth of Heritage: 'le moment Guizot.'" *Oxford Art Journal* 11, no. 2 (1998): 40–56. https://doi.org/10.1093/oxartj/11.2.40.

Poulot, Dominique. "Les musées d'histoire et la conscience nationale." In *Archives et nations dans l'Europe du XIXe siècle*, edited by Bruno Delmas and Christine Nougaret, 189–213. Paris: École des chartes, 2004.

Poulot, Dominique. *Une histoire du patrimoine en Occident, XVIIIe–XXIe siècle. Du monument aux valeurs*. Paris: Presses Universitaires de France, 2006.

Prendergrast, Christopher. *Paris and the Nineteenth Century*. Cambridge: Wiley-Blackwell, 1992.

Ragon, Michel. *The Space of Death: A Study of Funerary Architecture, Decoration, and Urbanism*. Charlottesville: University Press of Virginia, 1983.

Ramette, Xavier, and Gilles Thomas. *Inscriptions des Catacombes de Paris: Arrête! C'est ici l'empire de la mort*. Paris: Cherche Midi, 2012.

Reddy, William. *The Invisible Code: Honor and Sentiment in Postrevolutionary France, 1814–1848*. Berkeley: University of California Press, 1994.

Rosanvallon, Pierre. *La Monarchie impossible: les Chartes de 1814 et de 1830*. Paris: Fayard, 1994.

Rosanvallon, Pierre. *The Demands of Liberty: Civil Society in France since the Revolution*. Translated by Arthur Goldhammer. Cambridge, MA: Harvard University Press, 2007.

Samuels, Maurice. *The Spectacular Past: Popular History and the Novel in Nineteenth-century France*. Ithaca, NY: Cornell University Press, 2004.

Schechter, Ronald. "Gothic Thermidor: The Bals des victimes, the Fantastic, and the Production of Historical Knowledge in post-Terror France." *Representations* 61 (winter 1998): 78–94. doi: 10.2307/2902948.

Schwartz, Vanessa. *Spectacular Realities: Early Mass Culture in Fin-de-Siècle Paris*. Berkeley: University of California Press, 1998.

Serna, Pierre. *La République des girouettes (1789–1815 et au delà), une anomalie politique: La France de l'extrême centre*. Paris: Champ Vallon, 2005.

Shaw, Matthew. *Time and the French Revolution: The Republican Calendar, 1789–Year XIV*. London: Boydell Press, 2011.

Shorto, Russell. *Descartes's Bones: A Skeletal History of the Conflict between Faith and Reason*. New York: Doubleday, 2008.

Shovlin, John. *The Political Economy of Virtue: Luxury, Patriotism, and the Origins of the French Revolution*. Ithaca, NY: Cornell University Press, 2006.

Shusterman, Noah. *The French Revolution: Faith, Desire, and Politics*. New York: Routledge, 2014.

Singer, Brian. "Violence in the French Revolution: Forms of Ingestion/Forms of Expulsion." *Social Research* 56 (spring 1989): 263–293. http://www.jstor.org/stable/40970542.

Skuy, David. *Assassination, Politics, and Miracles: France and the Royalist Reaction of 1820*. Montreal: McGill-Queen's University Press, 2003.

Spang, Rebecca. *The Invention of the Restaurant: Paris and Modern Gastronomic Culture*. Cambridge, MA: Harvard University Press, 2000.

Spang, Rebecca. "The Frivolous French: 'Liberty of Pleasure' and the End of Luxury." In *Taking Liberties: Problems of a New Order from the French Revolution to Napoleon*, edited by Howard G. Brown and Judith A. Miller, 110–125. Manchester: Manchester University Press, 2002.

Stara, Alexandra. *The Museum of French Monuments, 1795–1816: Killing Art to Make History*. London: Routledge, 2013.

Staum, Martin S. *Minerva's Message: Stabilizing the French Revolution*. Montreal: McGill-Queen's University Press, 1996.

Steedman, Caroline. "Something She Called a Fever: Michelet, Derrida, and Dust." *The American Historical Review* 106, no. 4 (October 2001): 1159–1180. http://www.jstor.org/stable/2692943.

Steinberg, Ronen. "Spaces of Mourning: The Cemetery of Picpus and the Memory of the Terror in Post-Revolutionary France." *Proceedings of the Western Society for French History* 36 (2008): 133–147. http://hdl.handle.net/2027/spo.0642292.0036.011.

Steinberg, Ronen. "Reckoning with Terror: Retribution, Redress, and Remembrance in Post-Revolutionary France." In *The Oxford Handbook of the French Revolution*, edited by David Andress, 487–502. Oxford: Oxford University Press, 2015.

Steinberg, Ronen. "Terror on Trial: Accountability, Transitional Justice, and the *Affair Le Bon* in Thermidorian France." *French Historical Studies* 39, no. 3 (August 2016): 419–444.

Steinberg, Ronen. "Trauma and the Effects of Mass Violence in Revolutionary France: A Critical Inquiry." *Historical Reflections* 41, no. 3 (December 2015): 28–46. https://doi.org/10.3167/hrrh.2015.410303.

Tartakowsky, Danielle. *Nous irons chanter sur vos tombes: Le Père Lachaise XIXe–XXe siècle* Paris: Le grand livre du mois, 2000.

Thibaut-Payen, Jaqueline. *Les Morts, l'Église et l'État: Recherches d'histoire administrative sur la sépulture et les cimetières dans le ressort du parlement de Paris aux XVIIe et XVIIIe siècles*. Paris: Fernand Lanore, 1977.

Thomas, Gilles, and Xavier Ramette. "La création et l'aménagement des Catacombes. Premier musée souterrain de France au début de l'Empire, sous l'égide de L. É. F. Héricart Ferrand, entre 1809 et 1815." *Napoleonica. La Revue* 10 (2011): 66–98. doi: 10.3917/napo.111.0066.

Thompson, Victoria. "Telling 'Spatial Stories': Urban Space and Bourgeois Identity in Early Nineteenth-Century Paris." *Journal of Modern History* 75, no. 3 (September 2003): 523–556. http://www.jstor.org/stable/10.1086/380237.

Turner, Victor. *Dramas, Fields, and Metaphors: Symbolic Action in Human Society.* Ithaca, NY: Cornell University Press, 1974.

Van Kley, Dale. "Christianity as Casualty and Chrysalis of Modernity: The Problem of Dechristianization in the French Revolution." *American Historical Review* 108 (October 2003): 1081–1104.

Verlet, Agnès. *Pierres parlantes: Florilège d'épitaphes parisiennes du Moyen Age à la fin du XVIIIe siècle.* Paris: Commission des travaux historiques, 2000.

Vidler, Anthony. "The Paradoxes of Vandalism: Henri Grégoire and the Thermidorian Discourse on Historical Monuments." In *The Abbé Grégoire and his World,* edited by Jeremy Popkin and Richard Popkin, 129–156. Dordecht: Kluwer, 2000.

Vincent-Buffault, Anne. *A History of Tears: Sensibility and Sentimentality in France.* Hampshire: Macmillan, 1991.

Vovelle, Michel. *Le Mort et l'Occident de 1300 à nos jours.* Paris: Gallimard, 1983.

Wahnich, Sophie. *In Defense of the Terror: Liberty or Death in the French Revolution.* Translated by David Fernbach. New York: Verso, 2012.

Whitcombe, Edward A. "Napoleon's Prefects." *American Historical Review* 79, no. 4 (October 1974): 1089–1118. https://doi.org/10.1086/ahr/79.4.1089.

Woloch, Isser. *The New Regime: Transformations in the French Civic Order, 1789–1820s.* New York: W. W. Norton, 1994.

Wrigley, Richard, and Matthew Kraske, eds. *Pantheons: Transformations of a Monumental Idea.* London: Ashgate, 2004.

Zizek, Joseph. "'Plum de Fer': Louis-Marie Prudhomme Writes the French Revolution." *French Historical Studies* 26, no. 4 (fall 2003): 619–660. https://doi.org/10.1215/00161071-26-4-619.

INDEX

CPSIA information can be obtained
at www.ICGtesting.com
Printed in the USA
LVHW111956250419
615554LV00005B/119/P